GREEK AND ROMAN
MEDICINE

T0316234

Current and forthcoming titles in the Classical World Series

Classical World Series

GREEK AND ROMAN MEDICINE

Helen King

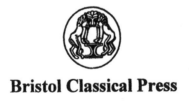

Bristol Classical Press

General Editor: John H. Betts
Series Editor: Michael Gunningham

This impression 2006
First published in 2001 by
Bristol Classical Press
an imprint of
Gerald Duckworth & Co. Ltd.
90-93 Cowcross Street, London EC1M 6BF
Tel: 020 7490 7300
Fax: 020 7490 0080
inquiries@duckworth-publishers.co.uk
www.ducknet3D631k

A catalogue record for this book is available
from the British Library

ISBN 1 85399 545 2

Contents

List of Illustrations

Acknowledgements

I would like to thank the staff at Bristol Classical Press for bearing with me, and my students on the 'Medicine and Society in Classical and Renaissance Europe' option at Reading for asking awkward questions. I owe much to the comments of my colleagues on an earlier draft of the manuscript: in particular, to Louise Cilliers, Philip van der Eijk, Mark Geller, Ann Ellis Hanson, Manfred Horstmanshoff, Edward James, Nigel King, Freek Rijkels, Frans Schlesinger and Marten Stol. The ideal working environment for completing this manuscript was provided by the Netherlands Institute for Advanced Studies, and Heather Ercilla at the Medical Photographic Library of the Wellcome Trust helped with the illustrations.

Preface

In all human societies, people have felt ill, and have tried to find explanations for their symptoms and ways of feeling better. Underneath these common experiences, however, there are many historical differences; for example, in how the body is thought to work, what is believed to be responsible for illness, how disease is treated, and by whom. We regard the Greeks and Romans as our ancestors in many aspects of our culture and traditions, and the great physicians of antiquity – most importantly, Hippocrates and Galen – are still honoured as medical heroes. But would the Greek and Roman experience of medicine have been much like our own, or something very different? In this book, I will suggest some of the similarities and the differences between medicine in ancient and modern societies and, in the process, investigate what 'medicine' is about.

Over its history, western medicine has had very obvious debts to classical culture. The treatises attributed to the most famous doctor of antiquity, Hippocrates, were translated from Greek into French in the mid-nineteenth century by a practising doctor, Emile Littré, with the intention of making real improvements in contemporary medical practice. A number of Hippocratic treatises, particularly one called *Aphorisms* which gives brief and memorable sentences on medicine, were used in medical education in Europe from the Middle Ages onwards; candidates being examined for a medical degree in late eighteenth-century Edinburgh still had to write about a Hippocratic aphorism. The 'Hippocratic Oath' is not universally sworn by doctors today (although many people still believe it is), but the need for an oath continues to be discussed by professional medical associations, and new versions which have been proposed by groups such as the British Medical Association are modelled on the Hippocratic original (see Chapter 2).

So what counts as 'medicine'? When we think of 'medicine', our first thought may be that this is something doctors do. We are all experienced in 'going to the doctor', that set of relationships which begins with a call to the receptionist, moves through an appointment consisting of a conversation and perhaps a physical examination, and often ends with a prescription and a visit to the chemist. In more serious cases, we may go directly to a hospital. In the ancient world, 'going to the doctor' was rarely possible; although, by the Hellenistic period, some cities had a 'city physician', those outside urban centres would probably never come across anyone who claimed to be a doctor, unless a travelling physician happened to pass by. In classical antiquity hospitals were only found in Roman military settings, or set up to treat sick slaves on a large estate. Some people would spend time at a temple of the healing god Asclepius, but these were places of pilgrimage rather than hospitals.

The criteria for 'being a doctor' may seem very different today. Medicine has become an institution, with state funding, in which education and licensing are strictly controlled. In contrast, in much of the classical Greco-Roman world there was no formal medical training. Even with our society's careful attempts to regulate medicine, however, we remain worried about it. We share cultural myths about doctors, which reflect our dependence on them as much as our fear that they know intimate details about our bodies and may reveal these to others. Until the computer-generated prescription, we laughed about the stereotype of the doctor with illegible handwriting, while avidly reading newspaper items in which this was blamed for the death of a patient. Stories of doctors who persuade a patient to alter a will in the doctor's favour, and then use their knowledge of drugs to murder the patient, horrify us, and suggest our unease at having to rely on medicine when we are too weak to do anything else. Fears concerning doctors and bitter jokes about their competence – or lack of it – were a feature of the classical world as well as of our own day (see, for example, Chapter 5): 'Trust me, I'm a doctor,' is still a phrase which elicits a wry smile. Today, the doctor uses appearance and 'bedside manner' to promote trust in his or her competence; the image of the white coat, with a stethoscope around the neck symbolising medicine's ability to detect what is hidden inside the body, is alive and well in hospital settings. The Hippocratic treatise *On Decorum* tried to encourage trust by advising the healer to act like a gentleman, dressing modestly, avoiding strong perfumes, and refraining from quoting from the poets at the patient's bedside.

Another area of enormous difference lies in the scientific underpinning of medicine. Surgical techniques improved from the eighteenth century onwards, with the status of surgeons increasing in proportion; germ theory was developed from the work of Louis Pasteur in the nineteenth century. The 1940s, when antibiotics were first produced, are often cited as the decade when – for the first time in human history – visiting a doctor actually improved your chances of survival. Medicine now has advanced techniques for looking inside the body: X-rays and ultrasound scans are basic tools in its armoury, while biochemical tests of blood and urine work at a microscopic level of the body that has only been explored from around 1850 onwards.

Does this automatically mean that medicine today is always more effective than the medicine of the past? Those who used ancient medicine, too, thought that it worked; efficacy could rely on experience of treating other cases, or on logical argument, but medicine still had a set of principles to guide what was done. In a fundamental way, the role of the doctor has not changed: he or she is continues to be the one who transforms a vague set of symptoms into 'a disease'. This can give the patient the reassurance that the symptoms are not unique but are something which has affected other people, which has an explanation, and which can be treated. It can often be reassuring to be told by a doctor that your illness is 'a virus' or 'something going round' rather than feeling that your suffering is exclusive to you.

In our medical system, 'going to the doctor' is not only about feeling better. We believe that illness is a valid reason for time off work, and an explanation for under-performance, so that emerging from the surgery with a medical certificate can be an affirmation that this is a genuine illness rather than mere malingering. Naming a disease is significant here: 'upper respiratory tract infection' sounds a lot better when phoning in sick than 'sore throat and a cough': 'pneumonia' is even more impressive as a label, but is hardly comforting to the patient. Being referred on to a hospital appointment may be terrifying or may be comforting, as a sign of being taken seriously.

The language of medicine has, however, changed significantly. In the classical world the words used by doctors were those familiar to ordinary people, or – where special names for parts of the body were needed – they were based on everyday language (see further Chapter 4). From the late medieval period onwards, when western European medical training was based in the universities, in which Latin was the language of instruction, doctors have been expected to know – or at least to use – some Latin. Many phrases and abbreviations used in medical case-notes and on prescriptions are still in Latin; for example, 'per cutem' for 'through the skin', and 't.d.s' for 'ter die sumendum', 'to be taken three times a day'. Many terms for symptoms and diseases now used by doctors are based on a mixture of Greek and Latin terminology, in which a muscular pain is 'myalgia' (which literally means simply 'a pain in the muscle'), and a spasmodic lower bowel pain is 'proctalgia fugax' (which literally means just 'a fleeting pain in the rectum'). These classically-based terms which doctors use can be baffling to ordinary people, but may be helpful as a further way of maintaining our belief in doctors as highly-trained professionals whom we can trust.

Medicine is also something that happens without consulting doctors. When we feel ill, our first response may be to excavate the back of the bathroom cupboard, to talk to a friend or family member, or to check a dictionary of symptoms. Depending on what we hear or discover, we may then speak to a pharmacist or browse the shelves of the local health-food shop. We may mix and match, visiting the doctor for a certificate giving our symptoms a name, taking the prescribed medication, but also paying a homeopath, osteopath or herbalist for other treatments. Where none of the experts seems able to make us feel better, we may join a self-help group of fellow-sufferers, surf the Web for information on our condition or seek religious healing by prayer or pilgrimage. In the ancient world, too, it was possible to treat oneself or to be treated by another member of the family, to combine different types of healing, to seek help in a temple or by using magic. There is much evidence to suggest that information about the body and about remedies was part of the general knowledge which educated members of the society were expected to share; encyclopaedias of the early Roman empire included material about health and disease.

Although it is a universal experience, therefore, illness exists in specific social and cultural contexts. This book introduces the topic of Greek and Roman medicine through a series of important themes, including developments in anatomical knowledge and new medical theories, while making suggestions about how we can locate medicine within the changing social contexts of the ancient world. It will also look at the fortunes of ancient medicine in later Western culture, investigating both the survival of Greek and Roman ideas, and the different challenges to their authority.

Chapter 1
The origins of Greek medicine

In the most general sense suggested in the Preface, medicine has always existed. People feeling unwell, according to whatever counts as 'well' in their society, have looked for explanations of their suffering and investigated how they could feel better. In the process they have developed theories to explain how their bodies work, and to assign blame for illness to internal processes – such as excess bile, or an 'upset' stomach – or to external agencies – such as gods, spirits, witches, the air, or germs.

Knowing the insides

Today, we are familiar with the illustrations of the interior of the body found as diagrams in modern medical textbooks, or in three-dimensional plastic models, so we tend to think that the skeleton and the internal organs form the basics of the body. In ancient medicine, however, just as important as solid bones and organs were fluids, for which the main organs acted as containers. Variations on this view dominated medical thinking until the eighteenth century.

The word 'anatomy' comes from the Greek language and simply means 'cutting up' or 'separating', for whatever purpose. But human dissection was not practised until third-century BC Alexandria (a historical hiccup which will be discussed in Chapter 4). This does not mean that people were ignorant about the inside of the body; on the contrary, 'cutting up' during animal sacrifice and butchery meant that the alignment of internal organs was well known from a very early date, at least for animals. The ancient Etruscans produced images of the human intestines to dedicate to their healing gods, although models giving such detail about internal organs are not commonly found in other early Mediterranean societies. Ideas about human anatomy relied on a mixture of animal analogies and chance. Aristotle dissected animals, and then made assumptions about people based on what he saw and on his belief that the human being was at the peak of the natural world. In early Greek medical writings we also find 'imaginary dissection', where a writer speculates 'if you were to do this, you would see that'; and there is a certain amount of 'accidental dissection', when the internal organs become visible through a wound or incision.

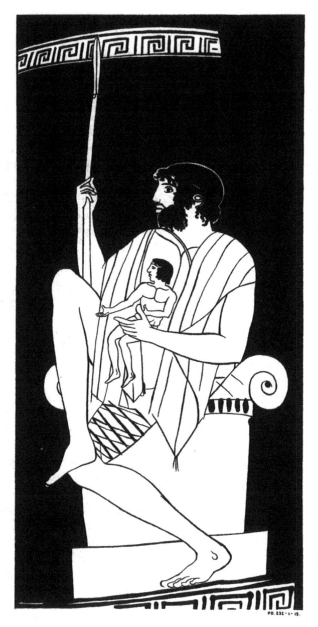

Fig 1 The hero Telephus, wounded in the thigh by Dionysus, holds Orestes. The wound was eventually healed by Achilles' spear. Coloured line drawing after an Attic cup, c.450 BC.

Wounds were a subject on which the early Greek medical writers were expert: they wrote books on joints, dislocations and fractures, discussing which were most difficult to set and outlining the different methods of bandaging. The earliest Greek literary work, Homer's *Iliad*, contains accounts of many wounds inflicted on the heroes who fought in the Trojan War; but when heroes such as Odysseus and Glaucus were wounded in battle or in hunting, their bleeding was stopped by a combination of bandages and incantations, or simply by the god Apollo.

Gods and disease

It is also Apollo who is responsible for one of the most famous diseases in ancient Greek writing: the plague afflicting the Greek army with which the *Iliad* opens. This is a punishment for Agamemnon's refusal to accept the ransom offered by the priest Chryses in exchange for his beautiful daughter. Homer sees the plague as the result of Apollo's sharp arrows raining down on the Greek camp. Apollo's twin sister, Artemis, shot her own arrows to cause disease in women. But not all diseases were seen as coming directly to individual sufferers from angry gods: in Hesiod's poetry, dating to around 750 BC, diseases are among the specifically human experiences which mark the end of the Golden Age when men and gods lived together. They were created because of Zeus' anger against Prometheus; they are one of the 'evils' released when the first woman, Pandora, opened the forbidden jar. Diseases then went on to wander the world in silence, afflicting humans by day and by night, but acting spontaneously rather than at Zeus' express command. Myth suggests that, whether sent directly by a god or part of what it means to live in the human world, disease is something outside our control.

The Greeks and Romans believed that the gods could not only cause, but also cure disease. Many gods included healing among their functions; worshippers left images of the afflicted parts of their bodies at shrines, and put up inscriptions describing how the god had helped them.

Asclepius

The most famous healing god of antiquity was Asclepius, son of Apollo himself. First venerated as a hero, at some point in the fifth century BC he was recognised as a god. The document known as the Hippocratic *Oath* (see Chapter 2) opens 'I swear by Apollo the doctor and Asclepius and the goddesses Health and All-heal and all the gods and goddesses...'. According to the standard version of the myth, told by poets such as Pindar and Ovid, Asclepius' mother Coronis was killed by Apollo, because the god was jealous that she had agreed to marry a mortal man. Her unborn child, Asclepius, was however spared; Apollo took him from his mother's womb on her funeral pyre and sent him to be brought up by the wise centaur, Chiron. Asclepius learned from Chiron about the powers of herbs and incantations, and also became a skilled surgeon. Chiron is associated with other mythical figures, including Achilles, and his method of instruction not only gave knowledge, but also morality: 'he trained doctors, guided musicians, and made upright men' (PHILOSTRATUS, *Heroicus* 9), and was known as the 'most virtuous' of the centaurs. However, this pupil went too far; Asclepius did not just heal the sick but, in some versions of the myth, he also raised the dead to life, using the blood from the right side of the Gorgon. Angry at this challenge to the boundaries between mortal men and the immortal gods – or, spurred on by Hades who complained that his role as Lord of the Underworld was becoming less prestigious because there were less dead people since Asclepius started work – Zeus killed Asclepius with a thunderbolt. The sons of Asclepius, Machaon and Podalirius, continued his work, serving in Agamemnon's army in the Trojan War (HOMER, *Iliad* 2.729-733). Later commentators on Homer suggested that Machaon specialised in the surgical treatment of wounds, and his brother in using diet; today, the brothers appear as the supporters of the Arms of the Royal College of Surgeons.

Some ancient sources suggest that Asclepius' crime was not so much raising the dead, but doing it because he was offered a substantial amount of gold as a bribe: this version of the story, found particularly in Christian writers such as Clement of Alexandria and Tertullian, is connected to wider concerns about having to pay doctors for their help.

At the temples of Asclepius which flourished all over the ancient Mediterranean well into the Christian era, patients made offerings to the god in the hope of a cure, or in thanks for having received one. The most famous sanctuary of Asclepius was set up around 500 BC at Epidauros; inscriptions survive dating back to the fourth century BC. There were also two sanctuaries in Athens. One is on the Acropolis and an inscription dates its origins to 420/419. The god was brought to Athens on the initiative of a man called Telemachos, who set up the sanctuary 'at his own expense', but it is not clear whether this was set up before or after the second sanctuary, located in the Piraeus port. To bring the cult to Athens, it seems that it was necessary to move a cult object from another sanctuary: in this case the famous snakes of Asclepius. When the cult was introduced to Rome in 291 BC, it was again one of the snakes which had to be moved to Rome to establish the presence of the god.

The snake was one of the animals associated with Asclepius and it soon became a symbol of the art of medicine. It was associated with immortality because it could renew itself by shedding its skin. Some accounts of temple healing involve these snakes licking parts of a patient's body; one inscription tells how a snake licked a sore on the toe of a sleeping patient. At Epidauros patients would sleep on the premises

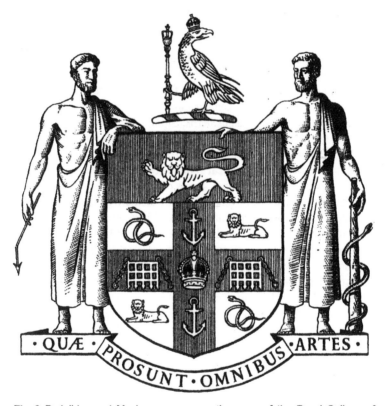

Fig 2 Podalirius and Machaon appear on the arms of the Royal College of Surgeons, England.

– a practice known as 'incubation' – where they would have dreams in which the god came to them and either healed them or advised them what to do if they wanted to be cured. Some of this advice is dietary, with the god advising a patient to eat particular foods or avoid others. In other cases the god gave recipes for salves or ointments to be applied externally. Some shrines of Asclepius also owned surgical instruments, so it seems likely that the priests would have used these on pilgrims.

Religion and medicine

The practices of temple medicine again show how close medicine and religious healing were in antiquity. We know of some doctors who worked as interpreters of the dreams of those 'incubating' in the temples of Asclepius; others were priests of the god, or contributed money to building and repairing temples. Inscriptions from some Greek sites in Asia Minor imply that, there, disease was sometimes seen as a punishment, and a gift was made so that the offended god would forgive the patient; sometimes the disease could be sent into an animal so that it would leave the patient alone. Hyginus' summary of the origins of medicine – a section which dates to the second-century AD or later – claimed that 'Chiron the centaur, son of Saturn, first instituted the medical art of surgery using herbs; Apollo first practised the art of treating eyes; and, in third place, Asclepius, son of Apollo, began the art of "bedside" medicine' (*Fabulae* 274). At the origins of the world as the Greeks understood it, mythical figures were thoroughly merged with what we would see as 'rational' forms of medicine.

These combinations of religion and medicine were not unique to the classical world. Early Egyptian medicine is known to us through the Edwin Smith papyrus, which dates to the seventeenth century BC but may be a copy of a text from a thousand years earlier; this lists around 50 case histories of surgery, mostly dealing with wounds, as well as giving incantations. The text is organised systematically, starting with the head and moving down the body. The Ebers papyrus, written perhaps a century later, includes a long list of diseases, many affecting the ears and eyes; the treatments it gives are a mixture of recipes, and magical incantations. The Chester Beatty VI papyrus is more recent – around 1200 BC – and its contents include 41 remedies for diseases of the anus. We also know that some doctors specialised in treating the anus. This is because the image of the body in Egyptian thought held that a series of vessels, called *metw*, carried fluids around the organs. These vessels started from, and ended in, the anus. Diseases were caused by *whdw*, 'rot', which came from the bowels.

From Near Eastern societies we have many baked clay tablets of medical content. From ancient Mesopotamia what is known as *The Diagnostic Handbook* survives. The earliest version dates to around 1600 BC and it had reached its canonical form by 1050 BC. This work forms a 'head to foot' arrangement of detailed observations of symptoms. The colour of the patient's skin and bodily fluids would be examined, so that the healer could account for disease by describing imbalances between four bodily fluids believed to be coloured yellow, black, white and red. But, while these cuneiform tablets show that diagnosis depended on factors which were directly visible to the healer, it was thought that diseases could be 'the Hands of the gods', and – as was done when demon possession was diagnosed – some diseases could be expelled from the body by using various rituals.

In ancient Greek medicine even the writers of the Hippocratic corpus thought that diseases had both natural and divine components. The author of a treatise called *On the Sacred Disease* criticises those who want to see each disease as caused by one particular god, and claims that they call a disease 'divine' in order to cover up their own ignorance of how to treat it. He himself ascribes the symptoms of epilepsy to an excess of white phlegm. When he criticises the name of 'the sacred disease' popularly given to epilepsy, he does not deny that it is 'divine'; he insists instead that it is no more 'divine' than other diseases:

> This disease seems to me to be no more divine than any other disease: it has the same nature as the others, and the same cause...there is no need to put it in a special category and to consider it more divine than other diseases; they are all divine, and all human.
>
> (HIPPOCRATES, *On the Sacred Disease* 5 and 21)

If it were truly divine, he argues, it could affect any type of person, but in fact it only attacks those whose constitution is already dominated by phlegm:

> Now, this disease attacks the phlegmatic, but not the bilious. Its beginning is while the embryo is in the womb, for the brain, like the other parts, is purged and develops before birth. In this purging, if it is done well and moderately so that neither more nor less than the correct amount flows away, the child has a thoroughly healthy head. But if more flows away from all the brain, and there is a great melting, then as the child grows its head will be diseased and full of noise, and will be able to endure neither sun nor cold.
>
> (HIPPOCRATES, *On the Sacred Disease* 10)

The parts and the whole

Thinking about how the body worked was not just a concern of myth and religion in the classical Greek world, it was also a theme of philosophical writing. The sixth-century BC philosophers known as the 'pre-Socratics' discussed the constituents of the universe, the basic building-blocks out of which everything was made. In the fifth century Alcmaeon of Croton defined health as balance, with all the qualities of the body – such as hot, cold, wet, dry, bitter and sweet – in harmony. He used the same word for balance – *isonomia* – as was used for equality of political rights, so that health became a sort of democracy and disease was a 'monarchy' in which an excess of one quality overwhelmed the others. Empedocles described the four elements of fire, air, earth and water, linking these to the four qualities of hot, cold, dry and wet; he claimed that blood contained a balance of all four elements, and that 'thought' existed in the blood surrounding the heart. Democritus thought that all things were made up of 'atoms', tiny and indivisible parts, in perpetual motion; in the debate as to how the sex of the embryo was determined, he argued that this did not depend on the temperature of the womb, with a cold womb producing a female baby, but was the result of the 'seeds' contributed by both parents.

Within early Greek society doctors were regarded as craftsmen. The Hippocratic treatises stress that medicine is a *technê*, a word somewhere between our 'art', 'skill' and 'craft', suggesting a skill which can be learned, with both a theoretical element – the 'why' – and a practical element – the 'how'. The *technai* were thought to have raised humans up from living at the level of the beasts and helped them to approach the immortality of the gods; in myth, Prometheus was thought to have brought the *technai* from the divine to the mortal world. The author of *Regimen 1* compares medicine with a range of other *technai*; for example, it is like the *technê* of the shoe-maker, because it cuts and sews to make something sound, and like that of builders, because it makes moist what is dry and dries what is moist, to create a harmonious whole. This very practical view of medicine also reminds us of earlier philosophy; medicine is believed to work with the different parts of the body to make a better whole and, in one of the few early sources for Hippocratic medicine, Plato said that Hippocrates thought the doctor needed to know 'the whole' before treating the patient (*Phaedrus* 270c-d).

Chapter 2
Hippocratic medicine

Seneca, writing in the first century AD, called Hippocrates 'the greatest physician and the founder of medicine' (SENECA, *Letters* 95.20). By the sixteenth century Hippocrates was being hailed as 'the Father of Medicine'. What are the main features of Hippocratic medicine?

The Hippocratic corpus

The sixty or so texts which are known as the 'Hippocratic corpus' mostly date from approximately 420-370 BC, although a few are much later. This group of very different early Greek medical treatises was brought together in Egypt, in the library of Alexandria, perhaps as early as the beginning of the third century BC. Some are substantial works, apparently by a single author; others are compilations of material; others are short pieces which may once have been part of longer works, now lost. Some give grand theories about the nature of the body and the origin of disease; others give recipes for remedies or advice on how to bandage a wound. The obvious differences between the texts, in terms of their origin, style, date of composition and the different theories they put forward, have been explained in a range of ways.

The myth of Hippocrates

The most popular way of approaching the Hippocratic corpus has been to try to link one or more of these very varied texts to the real Hippocrates. From antiquity until the late twentieth century the so-called 'Hippocratic Question' has been 'Which of the texts in the collection were written by Hippocrates himself?'. Yet we know almost nothing about the historical Hippocrates. A doctor of this name is mentioned in Plato's dialogue *Protagoras* (311b) and so, presumably, was active in around 430 when this dialogue was set and sufficiently well-known that Athenians had heard of him, even though there is no evidence that he ever travelled to Athens. Hippocrates is described as coming from Cos and as charging a fee for teaching people medicine. As both the island of Cos and the city of Cnidos, which lay opposite it on the coast of Asia Minor, were famous in antiquity for their doctors, one way of explaining differences in approach between different texts in the corpus has subsequently been to assume that some are from Cos and others from Cnidos. As Plato said Hippocrates was from Cos, this meant that medical ideas which were thought to be correct must be from Cos, while anything considered an inferior form of medicine was attributed to Cnidos.

In *Phaedrus* (270c-d) Plato adds a little more information, describing Hippocrates as 'of the Asclepiad family'. We have no contemporary evidence for Hippocrates' family but, starting with this description of him as an 'Asclepiad', writers in antiquity created a whole fictitious genealogy for him, which traced his family tree back to the healing god Asclepius and gave him several sons and grandsons who also practised medicine. According to this 'genealogy', and following a traditional Greek naming practice, his grandfather and grandson were also called Hippocrates, which conveniently meant that the less impressive treatises of the Hippocratic corpus could always be explained away as the work of someone else with the same name, or even another member of the family. From about 200 BC onwards writers also made up a set of fake letters – the 'pseudepigrapha' – in which Hippocrates corresponded with other historical figures, including the Persian king Artaxerxes and the philosopher Democritus. These letters were particularly popular in the early Roman period. Many long-lasting legends about Hippocrates can be traced back to them. One legend involves Hippocrates curing the famous plague which, according to the historian Thucydides, struck Athens in 430-426 BC (see Chapter 3): this story can be traced back to further fake documents created on Cos during the fourth century BC. The myths of the 'pseudepigrapha' envisaged Hippocrates refusing to help the Persians because of the enmity existing between Persia and Greece, and were later used in debates over whether a doctor's duty extends even to helping his enemies. Hippocrates replies to the Persian king's request for assistance,

> Send back to the King as quickly as possible that I have enough food, clothing, shelter and all substance sufficient for life, and I am unwilling to enjoy Persian opulence or to save Persians from disease, since they are enemies of the Greeks.
>
> (HIPPOCRATES, *Letter 5*)

It would be possible to argue that Hippocrates became the 'Father of Medicine' largely by default: he is simply the earliest Greek doctor for whom we have any information at all. However, another, more cynical view would be that it is the enormous range of views in the Hippocratic corpus that makes him such a convenient father. Anyone proposing a new medical theory will be able to find a passage somewhere in the corpus to support his or her ideas, and to give them the authority of the 'Father of Medicine'.

Hippocratic medicine

Although we know so little about the historical Hippocrates, we can still read the texts traditionally associated with his name. Known from early papyri as well as from manuscripts from the early middle ages, these works have survived because they have been copied; and they have been copied because they were thought to provide correct information on bodily processes, and effective ways to cure disease. What sort of works are they and for whom were they first written?

Because they date from the fifth century BC onwards, some of the Hippocratic texts represent our earliest surviving examples of Greek prose. Some look like public lectures, because they are written in the first person and seem to be arguing a point. Others may arise from teaching as they resemble lecture notes, or else take the form of simple, easily memorable sentences summarising particular situations. For example, *Aphorisms* includes, 'Pains and fevers happen when pus is coming into being, rather than when it has been already formed' (2.47) and 'When there is severe pain in the liver, if a fever comes on it takes away the pain' (7.52). *Aphorisms* was a key text in medieval medical teaching.

A further possibility is that the texts in note form were composed like a diary, in which a doctor wrote down anything significant so that he could go back later to think about it. Into this category fall the seven books of *Epidemics*, which record the changes in the condition of a patient from day to day; some passages even include the author's questions to himself, such as 'Is this the rule in an abscess?' (*Epidemics* 6.3.21). From the seventeenth century onwards *Epidemics* 1 and 3 have been the most favoured candidates for 'genuine works of Hippocrates', because their quality of careful bedside observation of actual cases was praised as being central to good medicine. The traditional title suggests to us a study of epidemic diseases but would be better translated as *Encounters*, because what is 'epidemic' here, in the sense of moving through a population (Greek *demos*), is in fact the doctor, as he travels from town to town. An example from *Epidemics* is:

At Larisa, a bald man suddenly had a pain in the right thigh. Of the treatments, none helped.

Day 1: sharp burning fever, he did not tremble, but the pains persisted.

Day 2: the pains in the thigh abated, but the fever was worse. He became rather restless and did not sleep; cold extremities. He passed a lot of urine but this was not of a favourable kind.

Day 3: the pain in the thigh stopped. His mind was deranged, with disturbance and much tossing about.

Day 4: near midday, he died.

(*Epidemics* 3.17.5)

Like the illness of the bald man, many of the diseases in the Hippocratic texts are types of fever. We would understand these as due to infections, the cause of which could not be treated with the knowledge then available.

The ancient doctor was expected to diagnose by studying the external signs in order to determine what was happening inside. Not only urine, but anything else coming out of the body, was examined with interest as a way of finding out what was going on in the mysterious regions inside. There were a few instruments which were used to enable the doctor to see into the body – for example, to examine the bowel – but, in the absence of X-rays, scans and blood tests, diagnosis usually had to rely on the patient's answers to questions and on what everyone could recognise through their senses. The writer notes that the bald man's extremities were cold, presumably because he felt his hands and feet for himself. Another Hippocratic writer notes of Philiskos, who died of his fever, 'his spleen was raised in a round lump' (*Epidemics* 1, case 1). Listening was as important as seeing and touching. In a case of lung inflammation, the doctor shakes the patient and listens to the sounds of his chest before cutting to let out the accumulated pus (*Diseases* 2.47); in another case of lung disease, it is noted that a sound 'like leather' can be heard from the lung (*Diseases* 2.59). Taste was also important: for example, 'Wax in people's ears; if it is sweet, it foretells death, but if bitter, not' (*Epidemics* 6.5.12).

In the case of the bald man, we can also see that the Hippocratic writers did not regard the mind and the body as separate areas; disturbances of one were believed to cause symptoms in the other. Elsewhere, madness was attributed to moisture in the brain. Too much phlegm caused epilepsy: too much black bile, melancholy.

In this case, the days of the disease are simply listed in sequence, but some Hippocratic writers believed that particular days were always particularly significant. Based on their experience of malaria, in which the crises occur on fixed days, they argued that other illnesses too had 'critical days' which could be survived if proper precautions were taken. It is not clear here why the writer chose to mention the fact that the patient was bald: did he have some theory in which it was relevant or was it simply to jog his memory when reading his notes later?

However, there is no way now of knowing whether any of the material of *Epidemics* goes back to the historical Hippocrates. The nearest to contemporary evidence that we have for his medical theories is Plato's claim in *Phaedrus* (270c-d) that Hippocrates thought the doctor needed to understand the nature of 'the whole'. This could mean the whole body, the whole of the patient's medical history, or the whole context of the patient's family and environment; or it could be Plato slanting the evidence to bring in Hippocrates as a supporter for one of his own theories.

Hot and cold, wet and dry

As we have seen, ancient philosophers were interested in the ultimate origins of all things and put forward different theories on what the basic constituents of the world may be. Most Hippocratic texts presented fluids in the body as the main cause of disease. The text *On the Nature of Man* names these fluids as yellow bile, black bile, blood and phlegm, known to later medicine as 'the four humours'; other Hippocratic texts talk about a different four – phlegm, bile, water and blood – or have only two or three such fluids, or regard the body as made up of fire and water. Health was evidence that the constituents of the body were in balance: disease showed that one had gained the upper hand. If a disease was thought to be due to insufficient heat in the body, then it could be treated with foods seen as 'heating'; exercise was also seen as 'heating'. The author of the Hippocratic treatise *On Fleshes* suggests that heat is the first principle: 'It seems to me that what we call heat is immortal, and knows everything, and sees and hears and knows all that is and all that will be' (*On Fleshes* 2). Later he states his belief that 'The most heat is in the channels and the heart, and because of this the heart, the hottest part of a person, holds the breath; this is easy to comprehend because the breath is hot' (*On Fleshes* 6).

Wet and dry were also significant categories in Hippocratic medicine. The treatises on women's diseases suggest that women are 'wetter' than men, with flesh of a more spongy texture that absorbs more fluid from their diet. This means that women were thought to need to menstruate regularly, or they would be swamped by the excess fluid and would become ill. The womb was seen as a collecting point for the blood, but it was believed that this organ could swing around and move up the body if there was not enough moisture reaching it. Because the liver was seen as a particularly moist organ, there was a risk that the womb would move up and attach itself to the liver.

As well as these oppositions between constituents of the body, Hippocratic writers used analogies between the human body and the natural world to explain what they could not see. For example, they suggest that the child in the womb is like a plant growing in a jar; if the jar is badly shaped, the plant or child will be unable to grow properly. Imagery from cooking and from agriculture is very common. Foetal development was seen as a process of 'mixing' and 'setting', in which the foetus is first like milk which rennet sets and then like a lump of dough rising in a warm place. These processes are followed by 'branching' as the fingers and toes are formed, and 'rooting' as the hair and nails appear.

In addition to creating balance between the constituents of the body, Hippocratic writers aimed to keep the individual in balance with external factors including the environment, the seasons, and the prevailing wind of the place where he or she lives. All such factors could interact with one's individual constitution. For example, a woman – who was by nature more moist than a man – living in a town with a wet climate would suffer from too much phlegm; her symptoms would be 'loose' ones such as diarrhoea and, if pregnant, she would run the risk of miscarriage.

The medical profession

To 'profess' is, in its original meaning, to swear an oath, and one of the most historically influential documents of the Hippocratic corpus is an oath in which a doctor swears aloud by the gods that he will respect his teacher and his apprentices, keep the secrets he hears in the course of his work and refrain from sexual relationships with the people he meets, whether male or female, free or slave. He also swears not to give poison, a clause which has been used in modern times as an argument against euthanasia, but which is better understood in the context of a society in which poisons and healing drugs were seen as dangerously close (see further Chapter 7). Another clause states that he will not give a pessary to cause abortion. However, this does not mean that Hippocratic medicine banned all forms of abortion, as in a different Hippocratic text a slave prostitute is encouraged to jump up and down to cause one (*Nature of the Child* 13). The writer of *On Fleshes* 19 also claims that some of his knowledge on the development of the foetus comes from observation of foetuses aborted by 'the common prostitutes'; he does not say how they came to abort. It is possible that some forms of abortion were thought to be safer than others, but it is equally possible that there was no common policy on abortion among Hippocratic doctors.

In any case, the *Oath* is in no way typical of Hippocratic medicine. We cannot be certain of its date – the parts dealing with the rules concerning apprentices may date before 400 BC and other parts later – or of the number and identity of those who ever swore it.

More commonly in antiquity, a doctor was not someone who had sworn an oath but anyone who claimed he or she was one, and who carried out medical treatment for a fee or a gift. Outside major urban centres the role of doctor was often not a full-time one and would be supplemented by, for example, land ownership. This lack of an exclusive identity was also the case with other types of healer, such as midwives. In the first century AD Soranus of Ephesus described the best midwife as a reassuring and sympathetic woman, free from superstition and not greedy for money. He also thought that she should have basic literacy and some knowledge of the theory behind her actions. This was clearly an ideal which could not be reached outside the larger cities; the normal midwife would have helped at a birth only occasionally, and we even know of one midwife in late antiquity who combined the role with that of bar-maid (EUNAPIUS, *Lives of the Philosophers* 6.3.6).

Far more characteristic of the Hippocratic texts is advice on how to behave to give the right impression. Doctors are advised to gain the trust of the patient and the patient's family by having a healthy appearance, a cheerful and gentle manner, and also by avoiding extravagant clothes and refraining from any discussion of fees when at the patient's bedside. Classical Greek culture institutionalised competition, from the Olympic Games to the Athenian theatre. In the Roman Empire we know that contests took place in the city of Ephesus in drugs, instruments, diagnosis and surgery, probably in public. The Hippocratic texts suggest that some treatments were performed in front of an audience: while the writer of *On Joints* describes how humpback caused by an accident can be successfully treated by shaking the patient on a ladder, he adds that this is sometimes carried out merely to make the crowds gape and stare. This treatment was also used to speed up a slow labour, although a case history in *Epidemics* 7.49 seems to blame it for illness in at least one woman patient: 'The wife of Simus, shaken in childbirth, suffered pain in the chest and ribs: cough, fevers, bringing up some pus.' *On Joints* also condemns those whose 'delight in pretty bandages' makes them bandage a broken nose more for effect than for the benefit of the patient; the bandages may look impressive but they do more harm than good. The fault may, however, lie with the patient rather than the doctor: the writer of *On Fractures* criticises patients who prefer novelties to tried-and-tested treatments of dislocated limbs. Healers could also work together; in the *Oath*, those swearing it say that they will treat their old teachers like their parents, and will teach medicine to their sons and to their teachers' sons without a fee. Swearing the oath 'by Apollo the healer, by Asclepius and by Health and Panacea' emphasises still further this tie between generations: Asclepius was the son of Apollo, while Health and Panacea (or 'All-Heal') were Asclepius' daughters.

The urge to take an oath may reflect the competitive social context in which ancient medicine found itself. Doctors were not only in competition with some other doctors: in their attempt to claim the authority to give medical treatment they were up against rival providers of health care, including family members, influential neighbours, root-cutters, midwives, wandering prophets, temple medicine and magicians. Even when the great Athenian statesman Pericles was ill in 429 BC, 'the women' hung amulets around his neck to help him (PLUTARCH, *Life of Pericles* 38). Ancient doctors could rarely fall back on their training to give them authority; there were no medical schools in the classical world and no exams nor professional licensing to prove who was, or was not, a competent healer. Some doctors would have learned their skills as an apprentice, often with a family member as their craft master. A few, particularly in the Roman empire, travelled the world studying with the famous doctors of their day, but there was nothing to prevent any persuasive person from attempting to cure others. The best way to gain a reputation as a good doctor was simply to treat a famous patient; in the second century AD, the great Galen (129-216 AD), the best-known doctor from the ancient world, cemented his reputation in Rome when he became personal physician to the emperor Marcus Aurelius and his family (see further Chapter 6).

Where it was a case of every healer usually being out for him- or herself, each would need to impress potential patients and sometimes – as in the situations described in *On Joints* – things could go too far. One of the techniques Hippocratic doctors used to gain trust was prognosis, using the present to predict the future. This helped the doctor to gain not only the confidence of the patient but also the faith of his or her family. In a famous passage prognosis is linked to the triangular relationship between the disease, the healer and the patient:

Speak the past, diagnose the present, predict the future; do these
things. Concerning diseases, practise two things – to help, or at
least to do no harm. The *technê* has three parts, the disease, the
patient, the healer. The healer is the servant of the *technê*. In
contending against the disease, the patient co-operates with the
healer.   (*Epidemics* 1.11)

Hippocratic medicine comforts its patients by claiming that the uncer-
tainties of health and illness follow a pattern, which can be understood
through careful observation: 'Nothing is random: overlook nothing'
(*Epidemics* 6.2.12). It gives an important role to Nature: 'Nature is the
physician in disease' (*Epidemics* 6.5.1). A number of other features were
taken up by later medicine as 'Hippocratic'; to different degrees, these
all idealise Hippocratic medicine or stress one treatise while ignoring
others. The main features singled out were the following: Hippocratic
medicine is free from superstition; it sets the patient in the context of the
environment; it is honest about its failures, never claiming that it can cure
everyone; and it is more interested in caring for patients than in making
large amounts of money, giving treatment to slaves and poor people as
well as to the rich. Each of these features can be given some support from
the individual ancient Greek texts themselves, but together they form a
legacy which is more than the sum of its parts, a 'Hippocratic medicine'
taking elements from very diverse Greek treatises.

Chapter 3
The Plague of Athens

In 430-426 BC Athens suffered two outbreaks of a mysterious, very unpleasant and often fatal condition, which still interests medical writers
today. The symptoms do not suggest bubonic plague, responsible for
later European pandemics such as the Black Death. Based on later
historical examples of 'virgin-soil epidemics' – diseases which have
become mild for one group, but which have a devastating effect on
another group exposed to the pathogen for the first time – measles,
smallpox, typhus, anthrax and influenza have all had their supporters as
culprits for the Athenian experience. Writers in the Roman Empire, the
Middle Ages and the early modern period all used the original account
of the 'Plague of Athens' as the basis for their descriptions of the physical
and social effects of epidemic disease. But how was this disease explained by the ancient Greeks?

Hippocratic explanations of epidemic disease

Some Hippocratic medical treatises proposed that disease was the result
of an imbalance between the fluids of the body, caused by a mismatch
between the individual – considered in terms of age, gender and constitution – his or her lifestyle, and the environment. The delicate juggling-
act of maintaining health was essentially an individual matter based on
self-awareness and monitoring external factors, altering diet and exercise
to make fine adjustments to the balance, and using more dramatic interventions such as fasting, purging and emetics where necessary.

For an essentially individualist system, epidemic disease could pose
a particular problem of explanation. How could many individuals, of
different ages and bodily types, all be struck with very similar symptoms
at the same time? One explanation was divine anger, as in the plague
which opens the *Iliad*. This could be shown by a dramatic natural event
such as an eclipse of the sun. The Hippocratic *Nature of Man* 9 argues
that diseases usually come from one's way of life, but suggests that
epidemics have a different cause. Whenever many people are struck by
the same disease at the same time, it is due to the air, since this – the
author suggests – is the only factor shared by young and old, men and

women, heavy drinkers and teetotallers, those who take a lot of exercise and those who do not, those who eat barley cakes and those who prefer bread. According to the legends which later grew up around Hippocrates, he and his sons cured the plague of Athens not by treating individual sufferers, but by burning huge bonfires to 'thin' the air. In his *Natural History* Pliny said that:

> Fire, even by itself, has the power to cure. It is well known that pestilences which are due to a solar eclipse are improved in many ways by lighting fires. Empedocles and Hippocrates have demonstrated this in many places in their work.
>
> (*Natural History* 36.202)

In other Hippocratic texts an epidemic disease can strike with different severity in men and women. In such a situation the air may again be to blame, but in the sense that men and women are exposed to the air to different degrees. In *Epidemics* 6.7, the description of a bad winter cough and fever which often turned to pneumonia includes the observation that free-born women rarely had the worst form of the disease, and the author notes 'I put this down to them not going outside, like the men'. Slave women, however, who would probably go outside the house more on errands, suffered from a particularly bad form of the condition.

Thucydides' evidence

Our sole contemporary source for this 'Athenian plague' is the historian Thucydides (*Peloponnesian War* 2.47-55). Born somewhere between 460 and 455 BC, Thucydides claims that he himself suffered from the condition but survived. In keeping with his view that the only valid history is contemporary history, the period for which eyewitness accounts are available, he described the symptoms and the effects of this condition in detail, so that future generations would be able to recognise it if it were to occur again.

However, doubts remain about the precise nature of Thucydides' graphic eyewitness account. If the Athenian plague was so significant in Athenian history, why do no other writers who were alive at the time so much as mention it? It is not included in Aristophanes' list of the evils of the Peloponnesian War given in his *Acharnians,* produced in 425 BC, although there seems to be a brief reference to it in Plato's *Symposium* 201d. In Roman history, there were a number of severe epidemics over the period 437-427 BC, which could fit with the general pattern of movement from east to west of epidemics in Mediterranean history. But, if this illness was such a significant event in the disease picture of the ancient Mediterranean, why is it not mentioned in the Hippocratic corpus, except in the later legends where Hippocrates is credited with curing it? For Thucydides, the plague was a very significant event in Athenian history; he attributes to it the loss of over 25 per cent of Athenian manpower, and states that it was the main cause of the decline of Athenian military strength (3.87). It may also have been responsible for the death of Pericles: Plutarch's biography states that Pericles only had a mild attack of plague, but it slowly wasted away his body and his spirit until he died in the autumn of 429 (*Life of Pericles* 38).

The plague as literature

The precise position of the description of the plague and its effects within the narrative of Thucydides' *Peloponnesian War* raises further questions. Thucydides places his account of the plague immediately after the funeral oration given by Pericles at the end of the first year of fighting. It is assumed that such an oration was given at each of the public funerals, held annually for the Athenian war dead, over the period of the war for mastery over the Greek world between Athens and Sparta and their allies from 431 to 404 BC. But Thucydides does not give any other funeral oration from the war; instead, he seems to compress them all into this first one, held at the end of the first year's fighting.

In Pericles' 'Funeral Oration', the glory of Athens is emphasised: the city is held up as an example to all Greece in the arts, politics and civic virtues. To move within a few sentences from this glowing tribute, to the horrors of the plague, looks like a deliberate rhetorical choice, reminding the reader that 'Pride goes before a fall'. This recalls a passage from one of Sophocles' plays, first performed in 409 BC: 'When one is without troubles, one should beware of disasters' (*Philoctetes* 504-6). In the overall scheme of the *Peloponnesian War*, however, the plague can have a further meaning for Thucydides' readers: so great was Athens that she was able to recover even from this disaster, and to continue fighting for another quarter of a century before falling to Sparta and her allies.

Thucydides' description of the social effects of the plague shows how near to the surface lie the forces of chaos and barbarism. He claims that one effect of the plague was the breakdown of normal funeral practices, with people even throwing corpses onto any funeral pyre they happened to find alight. Here Thucydides may be exaggerating for the sake of a literary effect, contrasting the order of the civic funeral for the war dead with the disorder of private funerals in plague-hit Athens; in fact, other literary sources include funerals and the erection of state tombs during the years when Thucydides says the plague was affecting Athens.

Explaining the plague

According to Thucydides, Athenians trying to make sense of the plague came up with many different explanations. Some believed it came from the gods, and therefore prayed, consulted oracles and visited temples; but, once it became clear that one was as likely to die in a temple as anywhere else, a lack of respect for the gods became widespread. Because neither living a good life, nor worshipping the gods, had any apparent effect, people came to the conclusion that there was no point in observing religious precepts. Here again Thucydides may be exaggerating, in order to underline his theme that neither the gods nor mortal men could do anything to stop this exceptional plague. The introduction to Athens of the cult of the healing god Asclepius in 420/419 BC – at the first opportunity, during the Peace of Nicias – suggests that some Athenians, at least, thought that the best preventative medicine was a new god. The purification of the island of Delos, sacred to Apollo, in 426 BC (DIODORUS SICULUS, *World History* 12.58.6-7), and the association of Apollo with the title 'Alexikakos' or 'Averter of Evil', also suggest that religious explanations for the plague continued to have power.

In looking for explanations, the Athenians thought that the disease had started in Ethiopia and had spread to Egypt, Libya and the Persian Empire before moving to Lemnos and then to Athens. This wide geographical spread was not consistent with Hippocratic ideas about local environments causing particular kinds of disease. However, Thucydides adds that nowhere was the disease so virulent as in Athens. Another possibility was poison: at first it was thought that the Spartans had poisoned the water supply in the Piraeus, but once Athens itself was affected this theory had to be dropped because the Athenian water supply came from deep wells rather than from more easily accessible reservoirs.

These types of explanation are found elsewhere in the history of disease. During the Black Death, one conjecture was that the Jews had poisoned the water supply. When syphilis first affected Europe in the late fifteenth century, each European country affected blamed its neighbours. For the English, it was 'the French disease'; for the French, it was 'the Neapolitan disease'. It was thought to come from the Americas, but its arrival in Europe was also considered to be divine punishment, delivered by means of an unusual alignment of the stars and transmitted through the air. 'Influenza' is so named for the 'influence' of the stars on this world.

Thucydides himself deliberately avoids speculating about causes, saying he will leave the question of the ultimate origin of the plague to later writers. But his account has suggested to subsequent readers that the reason why the plague spread so rapidly in Athens was the over-crowding due to wartime conditions. The Spartan army had just begun to maintain a base in the countryside outside Athens, so that the popula-tion of Attica was crowded into the city. It was the hottest time of the year and there was insufficient accommodation for the immigrants. According to Plutarch (*Life of Pericles* 34), the suggestion that over-crowding and heat were to blame was first made by Pericles' political enemies, who did not approve of his policy of moving the people of Attica off their land and into the city.

Medical historians reading Thucydides have suggested that he was the first writer to understand contagion, the theory that disease is spread by person-to-person contact. It was only in the 1860s that contagion theory defeated its main rival, 'miasma' theory, which held that the air spread poisons produced by rotting materials or stagnant water. Certainly Thucydides notes that overcrowding made matters worse, but this state-ment could equally well have been made by someone believing in miasma, as overcrowding and hot weather were thought to speed up the rotting process. It is interesting that, in the first century BC, when Diodorus Siculus was looking for a way of writing about an epidemic which struck a Carthaginian army besieging Syracuse in 397 BC, he used Thucydides as his literary model. On the cause of the outbreak, however, Diodorus moved away from Thucydides and argued that epidemics are sent by the gods, saying that the disease happened because the army had plundered the temple of Demeter and Kore. He added that it was made worse by overcrowding, the time of year, the heat, and the marshy, low-lying location (DIODORUS SICULUS, *World History* 14.70-1).

Elsewhere in his description of the plague, however, Thucydides makes other remarks which could be understood as showing an early awareness of contagion, although not exactly how it occurs. He notes that what caused most deaths was the fact that people caught the disease while nursing others suffering from it. This gives us some insight into how family members and friends were expected to bear the burden of caring for the sick, an impression confirmed by law-court speeches from fourth-century Athens. For example, in a speech from the early fourth century BC, a man tells the court how he cared for his adoptive father for many months, helped only by a male slave, losing sleep and suffering a great deal; the sick man's sister and mother came to visit, but the speaker expresses his surprise that no other relatives came to help out (ISOCRATES 19, *Aigineticus*, 24-8). Here Thucydides is not saying that nursing others 'spread' the disease so much as making the point that, because people became afraid to visit the sick, many died through lack of care. His second 'contagion' reference occurs in the introduction to the section on the plague, when he notes that mortality was highest among the doctors, because they were most often in contact with the sick. Again, this is only an observation: he does not go on to suggest the mechanism by which disease spread.

Medicine and the plague

Thucydides claims that doctors were unable to treat the disease, not because it was untreatable but because they did not know the right methods. Plutarch, however, who – like Galen – believed in the benefit of burning scented woods to counteract bad air, says that a doctor called Acron had some success in helping victims at Athens, by lighting a fire near to sufferers (PLUTARCH, *Isis and Osiris* 383 c-d). Reading Thucydides' detailed account of the symptoms, one can imagine any doctor being confused. The disorder started in the head and moved down the body, affecting in turn the eyes, mouth, voice, chest, and stomach. If patients survived the retching and vomiting, the disease went on to affect the bowels. Those who did not die could be left with the loss of their fingers and toes, blindness, or loss of memory. The sick felt such extreme fever and thirst, made no better by drinking, that they would jump into tanks of water if they could.

Some expressions used by Thucydides suggest that he was familiar with Hippocratic medicine. He starts his description of the symptoms with a general remark that the year was notably free from all other kinds of illness; this sort of comment on the general characteristics of a year is common in the Hippocratic *Epidemics*. He says that patients vomited 'every kind of bile that has been named by the medical *technê*'. He talks of the seventh or eighth day as the 'critical period' for sufferers, recalling the Hippocratic theory of 'critical days'. It is difficult to say whether other aspects of his description, such as the words he uses for inflammation, hoarseness and ulcers, are given in 'medical terminology', because the language of Hippocratic medicine is in any case so close to everyday language. But the overall approach of Thucydides – looking for patterns in symptoms, using individual experiences to build up a wider picture – is certainly 'Hippocratic' in the most general sense.

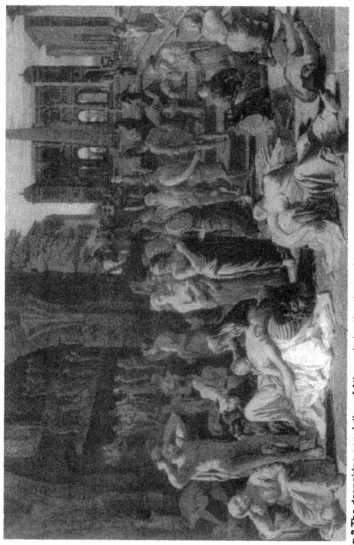

Fig 3 The despairing population of Athens during the plague. Line engraving by J. Fittler after M. Sweerts, London 1811.

The aim of Thucydides' account of the Athenian plague is not, however, 'medical' but 'moral' and 'historical'. He says that the plague led to selfishness, as people decided to spend their money on pleasure while they still had the chance. Considerations of honourable behaviour were abandoned, since no-one expected to live long enough to benefit from a good reputation. Crime increased because there seemed little danger of surviving to be brought to trial and punished. Those who survived the plague imagined that they were leading a charmed life, in which no disease could ever kill them. Thucydides emphasises in different ways the uniqueness of this event: its exceptional virulence, its appalling effects on individual sufferers and on the city of Athens. He suggests that a medical catastrophe can threaten even the mightiest state; that no human society should underestimate the speed with which a natural disaster can destroy its most basic values.

Nor was Thucydides the only Greek writer to use language close to that of medicine. All the writers of tragedy use medical images; characters suffer pain and insanity, while imagery of disease and cure is used for social disorder. Sophocles, who appears to have been personally associated with the cult of Asclepius, uses disease as a sign of heroic suffering: for example, the madness of Ajax or the poisoned foot of Philoctetes. These are not normal diseases; they are particularly 'savage', diseases fit for heroes, beyond what can be treated by human medicine. The intense madness of Ajax, which eventually leads to his suicide, is caused by the goddess Athena. In *Philoctetes* the hero is found suffering years after the snake bite which left his foot festering. He looks for herbs to help the pain, but it is eventually Asclepius himself who heals the sore.

Chapter 4
Alexandrian medicine

The great philosopher and scientist Aristotle, the son of a doctor, was engaged with his pupils on what they thought of as 'the enquiry into nature', an organised investigation into the whole of the natural world, including human beings, and a classification of what was found. Aristotle's enterprise covered everything from political systems to methods of reproduction. He was tutor to Alexander the Great, and the city of Alexandria, founded by Alexander in 331 BC, became the most important medical centre in the ancient world, maintaining this reputation even after the end of the Roman Empire.

Following the death of Alexander in 323 his empire split up, with Egypt being ruled by one of his Macedonian generals, Ptolemy. Ptolemy founded a royal dynasty and Alexandria became very wealthy. Much of the land in Egypt was classified as 'royal' land, while the king also took a share of the revenue from fees and taxes in all economic spheres. Imports were strictly controlled and attempts were made to run every aspect of the economy from an extensive bureaucracy based in Alexandria. Despite a near-crisis in the late third century BC, due to native revolts, some military defeats in Asia Minor and succession disputes, Egypt remained politically stable until the second century BC, with a Greek elite ruling the local people.

As part of a wider attempt to establish a place in the mainstream of Greek culture, the Ptolemies invested in patronage of the arts and sciences. Under Ptolemy's successors Alexandria became known for a strong interest in investigations into the natural world; the Library and Museum (literally, the Hall of the Muses) became an international centre of study. The aim of the library was to collect all the books in the world, and Galen and other writers preserve stories about how it acquired the hundreds of thousands of papyrus rolls it contained (one estimate is 700,000). Any book found on a ship docking at Alexandria would be taken to the library and kept, its original owner being given a copy. Books were also bought by more regular means, particularly from Athens and Rhodes, and some sources claim that the library of Aristotle's philosophical academy was among the works purchased. The Ptolemies believed that their role as patrons of scholarship was to encourage researchers as well as collecting books, and their patronage attracted philosophers, mathematicians, astronomers, poets and doctors from all over the Greek-speaking world.

Herophilus and Erasistratus

In medicine, the two best-known figures from third-century BC Alexandria came to the city in around 280 BC, possibly lured by the opportunities offered by the Ptolemies. Both originated from Asia Minor: Herophilus of Chalcedon (c.330 BC-260 BC) and Erasistratus of Ceos (c.330-255 BC). Herophilus is best-known for his work on anatomy, especially of the brain and reproductive organs, while the discoveries of Erasistratus were more in the field of physiology, or how the different structures of the body actually work. This distinction between anatomy and physiology, or between structure and function, is a little artificial, being based on much later ideas about the various fields into which medicine can be divided, but this only illustrates how our knowledge of all the ancient physicians is inevitably coloured by later medical developments.

An accurate picture of the interests of Herophilus and Erasistratus is difficult to obtain today because no complete work by either man survives. Extracts from their work are known only because later writers quoted from them, and even in these cases it is not always clear when someone like Galen is summarising (and so perhaps introducing his own ideas) rather than quoting the precise words of an earlier writer. In addition, Galen wrote treatises against the views of Erasistratus but generally approved of Herophilus. This means that we know more about Erasistratus simply because Galen found it necessary to say more about him, and his rating of the two men also slants the material he has preserved for us.

Herophilus may have written commentaries on the Hippocratic treatises *Aphorisms* and *Prognostics*, but also wrote a treatise entitled *Against Common Opinions* where he presented himself as a pioneer, rejecting what everyone else thought. He may have been both anchoring himself to the name of the great Hippocrates and stating his originality.

Herophilus' work on the brain and nerves is still famous because he rightly saw the brain as the centre of the nervous system and the base of the intellect. This contrasts, for example, with Aristotle, who gave the heart this role, but agrees with the author of the Hippocratic *On the Sacred Disease*, who wrote that 'the brain is the most powerful organ in the human being'. After seeing a functioning human heart exposed as the result of a wound, Herophilus decided that, because the patient still survived, the heart could not be as important an organ as Aristotle had thought. Herophilus' studies of the organs of reproduction revealed many structures not previously known; in the male body he identified parts of the spermatic duct, and in the female body the ovaries and Fallopian tubes. However, he did not know what these structures did; indeed, he may even have thought that the Fallopian tubes opened into the bladder. Whereas the Hippocratic writers thought that the womb was a special organ which could move around the body, Herophilus argued that it was made of the same material as the rest of the body and was affected by the same disorders. He gave the first detailed description of the human liver, accurately discussing its size, shape and position, while his studies of the pulse described variations in its size, strength and rhythm by analogy to music; he wrote of 'the music in our arteries'.

Erasistratus was the son of a doctor; the family remained a major site of medical learning. He is thought to have studied in Athens and on the island of Cos before working in Alexandria. His interests included the actions of the different valves of the heart. He saw the heart as a pump, with blood being made in the liver and going to the heart, with the arteries (carrying *pneuma*, or 'breath') and veins (carrying blood) coming out from the heart to the rest of the body. He discussed the process of growth, arguing that animals develop like a rope or a basket, with new materials being added on and taking on the same structure. Another process which interested him was digestion; here, he disagreed with the *pepsis* theory of digestion (the origin of the term 'Pepsi'), in which heat in the body 'cooks' the food, and argued instead that food was ground down by the stomach, stimulated by *pneuma* from the arteries. Unlike the Hippocratics, Erasistratus was interested in performing experiments to prove his theories. For example, he weighed a bird, then kept it without food. He continued to weigh both the bird and its excrement, and found that there was 'missing weight'; he concluded that the bird must be giving off matter invisibly. In general, he thought, the main cause of disease was an excess of blood overflowing from the veins into the arteries and causing inflammation. His main treatment was therefore starvation (so that less blood would be made); the obvious alternative option, letting blood by opening a vein, he regarded as very dangerous.

Both writers had to create new words for their discoveries, and they did this by using words which already existed, and analogies with processes outside the body. For example, Herophilus called one of the membranes surrounding the foetus in the womb the *amnion*. This recalls not only a word for a soft lambskin, so indicating the protective function of the membrane, but also a Homeric term for a bowl used to collect the blood of an animal which has been sacrificed, reflecting the idea that a foetus is formed from the blood of its mother. When studying the eye Herophilus called one of its 'tunics' or membranes 'net-like', from which we get our word 'retina', based on the Latin for 'net'. Words like these, still in use today, had a very different feel in their original context, where they related to objects found in everyday life and to beliefs about the body which we no longer share.

Dissection and vivisection

The discoveries of Herophilus and Erasistratus could not have been made without the opportunities they were given to study the human body. Later writers, particularly Christians writing under the Roman empire, accused them not only of having dissected humans, but also of having performed operations on people while they were still alive. Since even human dissection – let alone vivisection – is otherwise unknown in the Greek and Roman world, scholars have tried to explain why such practices could have been permitted, even encouraged, in third-century BC Alexandria.

Alexandria was a frontier city, where new ideas could be considered; Cos and Cnidus, where Hippocratic medicine developed, were in a similar position, on the borders of the Greek world and the Persian Empire. Greeks in Egypt would have become familiar with different cultural traditions about how a corpse should be treated. In Egyptian mummification, the abdomen was opened to remove the internal organs and the brain was drawn out through the nose. The separate organs were then put into different jars. Fifth-century Greek writers, such as Herodotus, found this repellent. In any case it was not the same as dissection for the purpose of gaining knowledge; Herodotus also implies that some forms of mummification just dissolved the internal organs, which would hardly be helpful for anatomical study. Greeks of the fourth century may also have had ideas about the relationship between the body and the soul different from those of an earlier period. If the body comes to be seen only an envelope for the soul, and a dead body is no longer seen as the 'person', then it may be less unpleasant to think of mutilating a dead body.

In practical terms it is possible that the patronage of the Ptolemies allowed behaviour which would have been impossible in classical Greece. We may assume that democracy fosters debate and is good for science, but in Athens you could be exiled if you spoke out of turn. In Egypt, however, the kings protected you if they happened to like what you did.

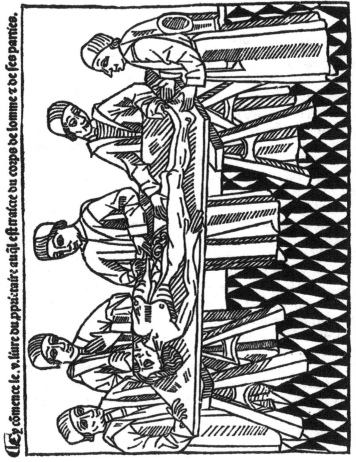

Fig 4 The earliest woodcut of a human dissection scene; line block after a woodcut of 1482.

Some sources even suggest that criminals and prisoners-of-war were supplied from the royal jails as victims. In the Greek world, torture was seen as a valid way of finding out the truth from slaves who were witnesses to crime and testing poisons on criminals was socially acceptable, so vivisection on such individuals may have been an easy step to take. The first Ptolemies did not try to integrate the Greek and Egyptian populations and may have felt that their Egyptian subjects were not fully human, thus putting them outside normal human conventions; an ethical move which, to us, is only too reminiscent of Nazi experimentation.

After the work of Herophilus and Erasistratus, Western medicine abandoned the dissection of humans for over 1500 years (see Fig. 4). The later kings of Egypt were not as strong politically as the earlier Ptolemies; it is also possible that traditional feelings about the unpleasantness of interfering with dead bodies were reasserted. Furthermore, a different medical approach developed in which dissecting people was seen as scientifically unnecessary, on the grounds that dead bodies could not reveal anything useful about living bodies; dissection did not help in understanding disease. This approach, which developed around 200 BC, was known as 'empiricism'. Empirics believed that the hidden causes of disease were not important; what mattered was effective therapy, and that could best be learned not from dead bodies but from accumulated observation and experience of which remedies had worked best in the past.

Chapter 5
Greek medicine at Rome

We know very little about medicine in early Rome. There is no Roman equivalent of the Hippocratic corpus, and before the first century AD all we have are isolated references from later literary sources together with some archaeological evidence, although few surgical instruments can be dated to the Roman republic. From the third century BC onwards it is clear that there were strong Greek influences on Roman medicine, but these were often found alongside a patriotic desire to present the earliest Roman medicine as something more simple, cheap and effective than Greek medicine. Greek medicine was presented as something done by outsiders for a fee: Roman medicine was performed within the family, based on the authority of the *paterfamilias*, the male household head. Greek medicine was seen as subject to constant changes according to fashion, while Roman medicine was traditional, stable and trustworthy. It is impossible to tell how accurate these caricatures are.

Greek doctors in Rome

According to the encyclopaedist Pliny the Elder, who compiled a guide to everything an educated Roman of the mid-first century AD should know, there were no 'doctors' – *medici* – in Rome before the arrival of a Greek doctor called Archagathus in 219 BC (*Natural History* 29. 12-13). It is not clear why Archagathus came to Rome; bearing in mind that he was granted the privilege of citizen-rights, it is likely that he was invited by the state. We know nothing of his training but he was welcomed with enthusiasm as a 'wound-doctor', an appropriate skill at a time when the Second Punic War with Carthage was about to erupt; Hannibal crossed the Alps in 218 BC. However, he may have come on his own initiative, looking for a new clientele. In this period there was considerable Roman enthusiasm for Greek culture, with Greek literary forms including epic, tragedy, comedy and history being adapted for Roman audiences. Archagathus was given a shop at a central crossroads where he could practise. However, according to our only source for this event – again, Pliny – he soon lost his initial popularity and was renamed 'executioner' because of his use of the knife and of cauterisation.

Another Roman source, virtually contemporary with Archagathus, suggests that Greek doctors were becoming familiar to a Roman audience at the end of the third century BC. Plautus' play *Menaechmi*, based on a Greek original, was probably presented in Rome before 215 BC, and features a comic doctor. When one of the two brothers called Menaechmus faints another character says, 'I'll go and get a doctor (*medicus*) as soon as I can' (PLAUTUS, *Menaechmi* 875). They have to wait for the doctor to finish his rounds, and he is hardly presented sympathetically: he has a mincing walk and moves 'at the pace of an ant'. The doctor asks the father-in-law what the diagnosis is: he replies 'But that's what we called *you* in for!' There is a complete lack of trust in the doctor's skills. The doctor asks questions like 'Do you drink red wine or white wine? Have you hardness in the eyes? Have you rumbling guts? Do you sleep well?'. These are very Hippocratic questions, although the diagnoses given are Latin ones rather than using words borrowed from the Greek language.

Not all Greek doctors in Republican Rome were so unpopular. In the late second century BC another Greek doctor, Asclepiades of Bithynia, set up a successful practice in Rome. Asclepiades rejected much of traditional Greek medicine, with its violent purges of excess humours and its surgical interventions. He believed that all disease was due to excess fluids or to blockages but also described 'particles' moving around the body. A blockage could even be combined with a flux, if blocked excess particles moved to another part of the body and then poured out by a different route. His speciality was gentle treatment: non-violent exercise (such as swinging on a suspended couch), food, wine, baths and massage. This contrasts strongly with Archagathus' use of the knife and the hot iron. But Roman medical tastes were not always for gentle remedies. Pliny attacks another Greek immigrant doctor of his own day, Charmis of Massilia, who persuaded people to bathe in cold water even during the winter. According to Pliny, even old men of consular rank would be stiff with cold simply to join in the fashion for Charmis' treatments (PLINY, *Natural History* 29.10).

One of the reasons for Roman unease about Greek doctors may have been some knowledge, and misunderstanding, of the Hippocratic *Oath*. Pliny claimed that doctors had 'sworn an oath together, to murder all foreigners' (*Natural History* 29.14). Plutarch mentions Cato's fear that Greek doctors have taken an oath but – echoing the story of Hippocrates' refusal to help the Persian Artaxerxes – suggests that the content of this oath is 'not to serve barbarians who were enemies of Greece' (PLUTARCH, *Life of Cato* 23-4).

Even in the Roman Empire most doctors continued to be Greeks; so, although some were citizens, many others were slaves or freedmen. With the exception of an elite doctor like Galen, the status of doctors in the Roman world was never high; like other craftsmen, they could belong to trade guilds which acted as social clubs and arranged banquets and funerals for their members. As had been the practice in some cities in the Greek world in the period from the fourth to the second century BC, some Roman cities employed 'public physicians', who were given privileges including various civic rights, immunity from taxation and military service, and a salary, although citizens would probably still have needed to pay them a fee for treatment.

'Roman' medicine?

Until Archagathus arrived, Pliny says that the Roman people lived without any doctors for over 600 years. Although he lived in a period in which Greek doctors were a familiar feature of the Roman medical scene, Pliny continued to believe that a medical profession was not necessary, because Nature herself has provided all the remedies we need:

> But Earth is kind and gentle and bountiful, ever a handmaiden
> in the service of mortals, producing by our forcing her, or pour-
> ing out spontaneously, what scents and flavours, what juices,
> what tactile surfaces, what colours!...she produces medicinal
> herbs, and is always productive on behalf of humankind.
>
> (PLINY, *Natural History* 2.155)

He considered that doctors were bad because they take away the responsibility for looking after your own health; if they are slaves, then it is even worse because they are reversing the natural social order by exerting power over free-born men. But living without doctors does not necessarily mean living without medicine and, in this self-consciously 'Roman', patriotic medicine, self-help was quite acceptable, as was medicine based in the home and administered by the family.

In keeping with their idealised sense of self-sufficiency, the Romans thought that the best medicine was very simple, based on a small number of ingredients readily available on the family farm, such as wool, eggs and cabbages. The main evidence for early Roman home remedies comes from extracts preserved from works by the politician Cato the Elder, also known as Cato the Censor (234-149 BC):

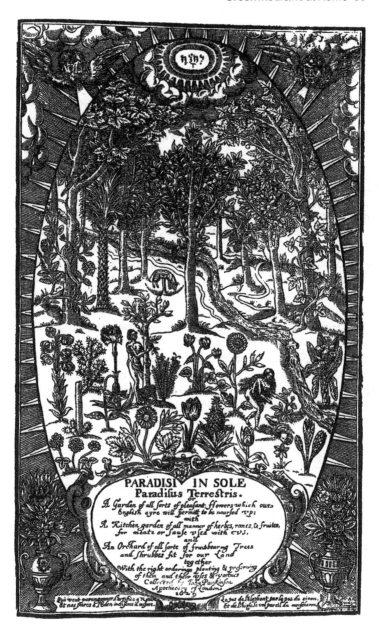

Fig 5 The title page to the London apothecary John Parkinson's *Paradisi in Sole* (1629) shows Adam and Eve surrounded by the plants given by God to cure all ills; a Christian interpretation of Pliny's views on the generosity of Nature.

The cabbage is the most outstanding of vegetables. It can be eaten cooked or raw; if you eat it raw, dip in vinegar. It is wonderful for digestion, and makes a good bowel movement; the urine [of someone who has eaten cabbage] is good for everything.... Wild cabbage has the most strength; it is necessary to dry it, and crush it finely. If you want to purge, the patient should not have dinner the day before, and in the morning – still fasting – give ground-up cabbage and a third of a pint of water. Nothing else will purge so well...

(CATO, *On Agriculture*, 156.1, 157.12)

The façade of distaste for Greek medicine could conceal a deeper level of similarity between Roman and Greek practices. Cato considered that Greek doctors could seriously damage your health; however, he admitted to skimming Greek books, if not to reading them properly. His praise of the cabbage could have come from a book on this vegetable by the Greek writer Chrysippos of Cnidos, which would make even this 'traditional Roman medicine' a thoroughly Greek product. The Roman writer Celsus included a book *On Medicine* in the encyclopaedia which he wrote for upper-class Romans in around 40 AD; the written sources he used were mainly Greek and he included references to a number of Greek medical instruments, such as the 'Dioclean cyathiscus' (literally, a spoon-shaped probe) invented by Diocles of Carystus in the fourth century BC, and used to pull out a weapon embedded in the body (*De medicina* 7.5). Even Pliny repeats many Greek herbal remedies, probably taken from Aristotle's pupil Theophrastus.

As part of his role as a household head Cato kept a notebook of remedies: some of these remedies, by which Cato treated his family, servants and slaves, were also incorporated into Pliny's *Natural History*. In his first-century BC work *On Agriculture*, Varro claimed that 'an intelligent shepherd can attend to the medical needs of the estate' (2.1.22) and suggested the chief herdsman could care for most diseases of workers and animals using notebooks kept on the farm, 'without the help of a *medicus*'. This is more a matter of economics than of charity.

At first reading, the surviving evidence may suggest to us that Roman medicine had more 'magical' elements than Greek medicine. For example, several medical writers of the Roman Empire cast scorn on the belief that hot blood from a gladiator's throat could cure epilepsy, but this only shows that some people used this treatment. Pliny tells us that 'Some people keep a weasel's heart in a small silver container, for swollen glands in a woman or a man' (*Natural History* 30.37), and that 'I find that a bad cold in the head clears up if the sufferer kisses a mule on the nose' (*Natural History* 30.31). Number magic was used (the number 3 was believed to be powerful), as well as a sort of 'homeopathic magic' in which, for example, putting out a fire by throwing wine over it was thought to reduce a fever. A famous passage from Cato's work, which includes two chants – the first using imaginary words loosely based on Latin, and the second in no known language – suggests that magical practices were used in traditional Roman medicine to cure a dislocation:

> Any sort of dislocation may be cured by this incantation. Take a green reed four to five feet in length, split it down the middle, and let two men hold it to the hips. Begin to chant: *motas vaeta daries dardares astataries dissunapiter*, and keep going until they meet. Wave an iron knife over them. When the two halves meet, so one is touching the other, take it in your hand and cut right and left. Touch the dislocation or fracture, and it will heal.
>
> (CATO, *De agri cultura*, 160)

This combination of chant and reed contrasts with Cato's comments on cabbage, where it is clear that the power resides in the plant itself rather than in any chanting accompanying it.

However, the apparently 'magical' nature of early Roman medicine may simply reflect the different types of evidence which survive; we have very little knowledge of how healing was carried out in the ancient Greek countryside. Magic also played an important role in Homeric medicine; for example, incantations were combined with bandaging to stop the flow of blood when the young Odysseus was wounded by a boar (HOMER, *Odyssey* 19.457-8). In the Hippocratic texts the role of magic was reduced, but objects could be used in a way which suggests that they had power in themselves. For example, an amulet to speed up labour is used in one gynaecological text: 'Smear fruit of the wild cucumber, which is already white, on wax, then wind up in red wool, and tie it around her loin' (*Diseases of Women* 1.77). Amulets using red materials were commonly thought to give a quick birth and one made of red jasper, showing the womb, has been found in Egypt. In Hippocratic medicine, although words had power the focus was on the persuasive rhetoric of the doctor, rather than on a spell which anyone could learn and use.

Chapter 6
Galen and his contemporaries

It would be impossible for us to think of medicine in the Roman empire without Galen of Pergamum (129-216 AD), the most influential and prolific of all the physicians of antiquity. He brought together earlier medical theories about the body, using philosophy to merge them into a synthesis which was all his own. Aspects of his work then dominated medical thinking until the seventeenth century. Most of his writings survive, many in Greek but some only in Arabic or Syriac. He wrote perhaps two or three pages a day throughout his life, and so has left us more material than any other writer in antiquity; we know of over 350 works by him, although many are now lost.

Galen was from the Greek East, wrote in Greek, and saw himself as a Greek. Rome was where he worked for much of his life but his heart remained in the Greek world, although he claimed to receive letters asking for medical advice from as far away as France and Spain. In his works Galen comes across as the centre of medical activity in Rome, and the target of malicious rumours by his jealous rivals. He tells us, for example, that some attributed his extraordinary success in prognosis to magical rather than medical skills. On one famous occasion described in his treatise *On Prognosis*, he detected that a woman's pulse rate increased when the name of the man she loved was mentioned. Galen himself attributed his prognostic skills mainly to following Hippocratic principles based on reading bodily signs and being aware of all relevant features of the patient's life, and he attacked other doctors of his time for failing to understand what Hippocrates really meant. He calls Hippocrates 'our guide to all good things' and says that, to find out if a doctor really knows about medicine, you should ask him where in the works of Hippocrates something is mentioned, and how Hippocrates came to the conclusions he reached.

Yet should we believe what Galen tells us? By telling us he is so good that his powers seem almost supernatural he is carrying on the Hippo-cratic tradition of self-promotion, while recalling healers of the past, such as Empedocles, who were credited with having been able even to raise the dead. His insistence that all he does is to follow faithfully what

Hippocrates recommended is a way of giving the authority of tradition to his actions, even if he is doing something quite novel. But this is rhetoric; the 'Hippocrates' Galen gives us is one created in Galen's own image. Galen's very personal judgements of which treatises in the Hippocratic collection were the 'genuine works' of Hippocrates have influenced all subsequent work on those treatises. The problem with Galen is that the survival of so much of his work makes us fall under his spell, entranced into believing that he embodied what the medicine of the Roman empire was all about.

A glance at Galen's biography – again, known from what he chooses to tell us – shows us just how far he was from being a typical healer of his time. Most healers, whose names and other biographical information are available to us from inscriptions, were small-scale operators, some specialising in a particular disease. Their training would be at best minimal, perhaps given to them by a family member. In the Roman empire of the second century, women as well as men could be doctors; a funerary inscription found in Spain was set up by the husband of Julia Saturnina, 'best *medica* and most pious of women' (CIL II 492 = ILS 7802). It is unclear whether a woman *medica* could do everything a male *medicus* was able to do; it is possible that a woman was only allowed to treat other women, children and slaves, so that a husband and wife team could divide up their patients between them. From second-century AD Ostia, we have a terracotta relief from the tomb of Scribonia Attica, who was a midwife; her husband, M. Ulpius Amerimnus, was a doctor and surgeon. The woman whose baby is being delivered sits on a birthing chair, supported by another woman, while Scribonia sits on a stool in front of her and delivers the child.

Galen's training and career

Although texts such as the Hippocratic *Law* 2 claim that students of medicine should ideally start their education in childhood, in the real life of the ancient world Galen's background of privilege and extensive training was unique. He was born in Pergamum, a former Hellenistic capital, part of the Roman empire since the mid-second century BC and the home of a famous temple of Asclepius. The son of a rich architect, he studied philosophy, but his father was commanded by a dream from the god Asclepius to encourage him towards a medical education. Galen began his medical career in 145-6; he started training in his home town but then, because his family was so wealthy, he was able to visit famous teachers of medicine at Smyrna, Corinth and Alexandria, and to continue his training for many years. By the time Galen saw his first patient, most doctors in the Roman world would have been practising for over a decade. From 157 he worked as physician to a team of gladiators in Pergamum, where he claims to have significantly reduced the death rate among those wounded in the arena, before moving to Rome in 162.

In this period Rome was a stable environment with a population of around one million people, providing opportunities for many doctors, even those with relatively specialised medical skills. For a rich young man with an impressive background, it was the perfect place. To impress the men who mattered at Rome, Galen continued to use skills which he had developed in Pergamum. In his treatise *On Examinations by which the Best Physicians are Recognised* Galen describes how he performed demonstrations on animals, removing and then replacing the intestines of an ape, in order to impress the other physicians and leading citizens of Pergamum; he continued to perform such public demonstrations in Rome.

However, although Greek medicine was by now part of Roman culture, with around 75 per cent of doctors in the Roman Empire coming from the Greek East, the idea that medicine was not really a respectable activity for a civilised man continued. Galen overcame some of this prejudice by using his own elite background, finding his first patients through social contacts of his father and of his own teachers. As he tells us proudly in his treatise *On Prognosis*, he was soon treating high-class patients, 'almost all the social and intellectual elite of the city of Rome' (*On Prognosis* 2). After other doctors had given up Galen treated the philosopher Eudemus for a fever, accurately predicting when the next convulsion would occur. Impressed with Galen's medical skills, Eudemus then told his visitors (Flavius Boethus, a former consul, and Sergius Paulus, who went on to become City Prefect) about Galen, so that his reputation spread. As part of his attempts to make the trade of medicine into a respectable activity for a gentleman, Galen insisted that that the best doctor is also a philosopher; this clearly helped him to win patients from the Roman elite. Both Eudemus and Boethus were, Galen tells us, followers of Aristotelian philosophy, as was the emperor's uncle Barbarus (who had been consul in 157 AD). Galen 'talked their language'.

Despite his successes Galen left Rome in 165, alleging that other physicians in Rome were jealous of him and were trying to damage his reputation and stop him from seeing patients.

His abrupt departure was, however, possibly due to an attempt to avoid the smallpox epidemic which hit Rome soon after. On his return in 169 he became doctor to the emperor Marcus Aurelius and his family, although he managed to avoid accompanying the imperial household on the dangerous campaign in Germany by claiming he could not go on religious grounds; Asclepius had warned him in a dream not to travel. One aspect of his role in the imperial household was to prepare theriac, a multi-ingredient, cure-all drug, which Marcus and many other members of the Roman elite insisted on taking: Galen's personal recipe included 77 ingredients, one of which was latex from the opium poppy. It was also used as a prophylactic, a drug taken to prevent illnesses.

The Galenic body

Galen believed that medicine required both practical and theoretical elements. He claimed that he dissected animals every day; usually Barbary apes, pigs, goats and sheep but, on one occasion, the heart of an elephant. Much of this work was done in private as practice for his public performances, where he even asked members of the audience to choose which part he was to dissect. He was aware of the fine line between impressing the audience, and horrifying them. He noted that the difficulty of performing experiments on the brain of live monkeys was that their expressions could be too 'human' for comfort, and instead recommended using pigs or goats for work on the brain; however, he also liked to use pigs or goats because they made a louder noise while the experiment was in progress. His experiments on the spinal cord, in which he demonstrated that muscles are controlled by nerves, are still famous.

However, all these experiments were performed on animals, particularly pigs and apes, rather than on humans. In Galen's version of the human body, some parts he describes do not in fact exist. These derive from incorrect analogies between animals and humans; for example, the 'rete mirabile' (literally, 'the miraculous net') at the base of the skull, which is not found in humans. Other errors, such as the 'invisible pores' which Galen insisted must be present in the septum dividing the two halves of the heart, were logically necessary to his model of the body. As we shall see in Chapter 8, it was not for many centuries that these errors were discovered.

In the Galenic body each part is created for a specific purpose, and heat plays a central role in the whole. The three 'faculties' of the body are, in ascending order of importance, the nutritive, the vital and the logical faculties. In the nutritive sphere – shared with plants and animals – food is partially cooked by the stomach into a fluid called chyle, and is then drawn via the portal vein to the liver, where it is heated further and the 'natural spirit' is added. Parts of the body 'attract' to themselves for nourishment most of the 'venous blood' which the liver makes. Some fluid, however, travels on by way of the vena cava to the heart, where in a further stage of cooking it takes in 'vital spirit' to become lighter and thinner, as 'arterial blood'. This transmits to other parts of the body the vital faculty, shared by humans with other animals, which gives warmth and the power of growth and can be measured through the pulse. The brain gives the blood psychic *pneuma* which is distributed through the body by means of the nerves; with the brain is associated the logical faculty: the power of thought, will and choice which is unique to humans. In contrast to the model of the circulation of the blood put forward by William Harvey in 1628, the Galenic body has veins, arteries and nerves as three separate systems with different functions. For Galen, any vessel which began or ended in the right side of the heart was called a 'vein', and any vessel connected to the left side of the heart was an 'artery'. For Harvey, however, veins and arteries formed one system centred on the heart, with the arteries carrying blood away from the heart and the veins returning it there again.

Although the fluids are the most important features of this body, the solid organs also have 'faculties' or powers. They can attract or repel, retain or expel. An organ can be too weak to attract the nutritive blood from the liver, but also the channels can be narrowed by obstruction, or the fluids they carry can be too thick and move too slowly, perhaps because the patient is eating the wrong foods. Illness can therefore be due to a fault in an organ, a channel or a fluid.

In the course of Galen's long life his ideas about the body changed, while the needs of the different audiences for which his work was written also affected how he presented his ideas. After his death his many works were used to construct 'Galenism', a far more systematised model of the body than that given in any one Galenic treatise. This model of the body combined ideas from Hippocratic medicine, Plato and Aristotle. The scientific logic is Aristotelian, while the notion of three body systems governed by the heart, the brain and the liver respectively comes from Plato, the fourth century BC Athenian philosopher whose dialogue, the *Republic*, divides the soul into three parts, namely reason, 'spirit' or emotion, and desire.

Galen adopted from the Hippocratic treatise *Nature of Man* the idea of four humours, or body fluids. For health these needed to be in balance. In Galen's thought and, to an even greater degree, in the work of later writers who tried to condense his enormous output into a more manageable structure, this became the basis of a far-reaching system in which each humour could be tied to a quality, a season, a period of the life-cycle, a time of day, a colour and a taste. Blood, the warm and moist fluid, was associated with spring and predominated in childhood; yellow bile was considered warm and dry and was associated with summer and youth; black bile, thought to be cold and dry, was associated with autumn and adulthood; phlegm, cold and moist, was the humour of winter and of old age. Healing, for Galen, involved the application of general principles to specific, individual cases. The maintenance of the correct balance amongst the four humours in any individual body constitutes health, while imbalances can be corrected by attention to air, food and drink, exercise, sleep, repletion and evacuation, and emotion.

Chapter 7
Curing illness

According to Celsus, after Hippocrates medicine became divided into three major branches: diet, drugs and surgery. These healing activities were not of equal status, even though the ancient doctor was normally expected to be able to use all three. Diet was the first line of action. In the fourth century BC, Plato (*Timaeus* 89b-d) suggested that, as far as possible, any diseases that were not very dangerous should be treated by diet; drugs would cause more harm than good, because they cut short the normal lifespan of a disease and this would lay the body open to more serious diseases. Surgery would be used only if all else failed. Those who swore the Hippocratic *Oath* said that they would not perform 'cutting', and would leave cases of bladder stone to those who specialised in this operation; however, other Hippocratic texts do not share this reluctance, and include surgery in the range of measures a doctor could employ. Galen, although he performed some difficult surgery, including the removal of the breastbone, suggested that a doctor should be most highly praised if he could cure all diseases without resorting to surgery (*On Recognising the Best Physicians* 10.2). Galen also recommended removing excess blood, which would move the other humours if they had accumulated in one place and were causing symptoms there.

Diet

Much of ancient medicine was based on diet in the original broad sense of the Greek word *diaita*, meaning 'way of life'. Galenic medicine drew attention to what it called 'the six non-naturals': food and drink, air, motion and rest, sleep and waking, excretion and retention, and the passions of the mind. These 'non-naturals' were the factors most closely affecting the natural state of the body and, if they were not properly managed, then a 'contra-natural' state of illness would be the result. Because food made the humours, any disturbance in the humoral balance could first be addressed by changing the diet. In the most sophisticated dietary texts of the ancient world, it was also necessary to have the correct diet for one's age and gender, and to adjust it further according to seasonal changes; in winter, for example, one should follow a dry, warm diet.

The Hippocratic treatise *On Regimen*, dating from the early fifth or late fourth century BC, is the fullest discussion of this type in the Hippocratic corpus. The author argues that children are warm and moist; young men warm and dry; mature men cold and dry; and old men cold and moist. Men are generally warmer and drier than women (*On Regimen* 1.23-24). In the second book exercise is discussed in detail, according to the time of day one exercises and how much clothing is worn. Seeing, hearing, speaking and thinking are included as types of exercise; for example, when sound strikes the soul, it is exercised, warmed and dried. Thinking has similar effects, so it can 'make a person thin' (*On Regimen* 2.61). Foods are listed by type – fruits, vegetables, meats and so on – according to their properties:

> Coriander is warm and astringent: it stops heartburn, and when eaten last it leads to sleep. Lettuce is quite cooling until it has juice, but sometimes it produces weakness in the body. Dill is hot and astringent, and its smell stops sneezing.
>
> (*On Regimen* 2.54)

Here it is very difficult to draw the line between 'foods' and 'medicines'. All foods have properties which act on the body, and must be considered even in health. The everyday food intake can be altered to heat or dry the body, to produce less phlegm or more blood, but it is also possible to 'prescribe' very specific substances outside meal times, or to have them administered externally. If a patient survives fourteen days of pain in the back, with fever and blood in the urine – in our terms, probably a severe kidney infection – he should be given millet for breakfast and boiled puppy or fowl in the evening; the instructions insist that he should also 'drink the sauce' (*Diseases* 2.56). Why should this be so important? Puppy meat is described in *Regimen* 2.46 as moistening and as passing very well in the urine, so it may be considered as the safest meat for this patient. This example seems to be closer to 'food' than 'medicine'. Another example is more complicated. When a patient suffers from a wound, he should eat nothing, drink only water and vinegar, and take a thin gruel. However, when the writer goes on to say that inflammation of the wound should be treated with cooling plasters containing boiled beets, celery, or the boiled leaves of the olive, fig, elder, bramble or pomegranate, then this external application seems to be using 'food-stuffs' as 'medicines' (*Affections* 38).

For Roman medicine, diet had strong moral overtones. Throughout Roman history, laws were passed restricting the use of gourmet foods.

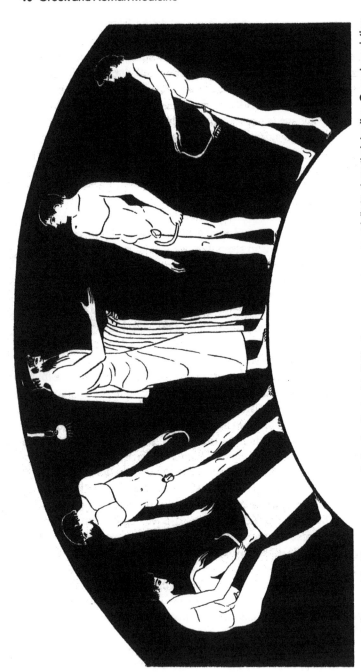

Fig 6 Exercise and bathing were seen as balancing the body's fluids; here, young men use strigils to clean their bodies. Gouache painting from an Attic kylix of the mid-fifth century BC.

Rich and highly-seasoned foods were thought to be very dangerous, and Roman moralists often exhorted their fellow citizens to return to the simple diet of their ancestors; baked turnip was seen as a particularly traditional, unadorned food. By the early Roman Empire, it was thought that contact with other nations – above all, in the decadent East – was weakening traditional Roman values of austerity and restraint. This included contact with new foodstuffs.

In Plautus' play, *Pseudolus*, a cook suggests that upper-class Romans had even taken to 'seasoning their herbs with other herbs' (*Pseudolus* 1.810). In the fictional banquet of Trimalchio, the dishes served included quinces covered in thorns to make them look like sea-urchins, and what looked like a goose surrounded by fish and birds, but which in fact was all made out of pork (PETRONIUS, *Satyricon* 69-70). Plutarch considered that 'it is the things that sustain life which also cause sickness' (*Table-talk* 731d); he listed honeyed wine and sow's wombs as new items on the Roman menu, while changes had also been made to the order of courses on the menu and to drinking habits. Pliny had earlier dated to the rule of the emperor Tiberius the fashion for drinking wine on an empty stomach before the meal, which he saw as a foreign practice (*Natural History* 14.143). Seneca too expostulated against the dangers of culinary innovation; once mankind started to devise a thousand different sauces, the digestive system gave up in disgust. Seneca announced that 'It is not surprising that diseases are beyond counting: just count the cooks!' (*Epistle to Lucillus* 95). The answer to this diet was to induce vomiting; as Seneca put it, 'Down with it quickly, and up with it quickly!' (*Moral Letters* 108.13-15).

Drugs

Some substances were not normally eaten, or were combined in a way which would not occur at the dinner table: these we may properly call 'drugs'. Some Hippocratic examples are: 'When this happens, give the patient to drink five obols weight of black hellebore, in sweet wine' (*Internal Affections* 48); 'Lozenge for pneumonia: juice of "all-heal" and pine-cone in Attic honey' (Appendix to *Regimen in Acute Diseases* 34). Some drugs were common materials in the Mediterranean region, while others were exotic materials imported from distant parts of the known world: Egyptian perfume, myrrh and narcissus oil. Some drugs were very famous; for example, 'Lemnian earth' which, according to Galen, came in three types, only one being medicinal. Used to stop wounds bleeding and to induce vomiting if poison had been taken,

Lemnian earth was taken from only one hill, on which no one but a priestess was allowed to walk, and it was stamped with an image of the goddess Diana (GALEN, *On Simple Medicines* 9.2). Lists of drugs for a condition often gave many alternatives, perhaps because not all would be available throughout the year, or perhaps so that the doctor could prescribe something the patient would be able to afford.

Whereas Babylonian medicine referred to some diseases as 'Hand of the god', for Herophilus drugs were 'the hands of the gods' (fr. 248-9 von Staden). As we have seen in Chapter 5, Pliny believed that a kindly Nature 'produces medicinal herbs, and is always productive on behalf of humankind' (*Natural History* 2.156). But Nature was also responsible for creating poisons. In the ancient world there was considerable concern about the line between what we would call 'drugs' and 'poisons', the Greek word *pharmakon* covering both. Diocles of Carystos – described by Pliny (*Natural History* 26.10) as second only to Hippocrates – wrote a lost work called *Rhizotomikon* ('Rootcutting') which seems to have listed plants alongside their medical effects; to him are also attributed works 'On vegetables' and 'On lethal drugs'. Some Hippocratic treatises mention a lost work called *Pharmaka*. It may have grouped drugs by their main qualities; for instance, at the end of the treatise called *Places in Man* we read very general advice to 'apply any of the foul-smelling substances you wish'; 'apply pleasant-smelling and warming substances'; 'apply warming substances' which include 'cow dung, bull's gall, myrrh, alum, all-heal juice and anything similar'; 'purge with mild laxatives'; and so on.

Sometimes the connections between a substance and its healing qualities are clearly symbolic; for example,

> An egg is strong, because it is the starting point for the creature; it is nourishing, because it is the milk of the creature; and it pro-duces wind, because it expands from a small size to a large one.
>
> (*Regimen* 2.50)

Many other substances used in healing had associations with myth and religion. In the *Homeric Hymn to Demeter* (210) the goddess Demeter drank a *kykeon* while she was searching for her missing daughter Persephone; this drink, made with barley, cheese and wine, and flavoured with honey or herbs such as pennyroyal, was also used extensively in Hippocratic medicine as a restorative. The herb *agnus castus* was used in the all-women ritual of the Thesmophoria, where it preserved the chastity of the married women involved during the ritual but encouraged their fertility once they were back home. It also features in Hippocratic recipes for women's diseases. Squill was used in purification rituals, where it drove out evil forces, and also in medicine.

In Hippocratic medicine, as the examples already given show, dosage was not always stated, but in the case of certain substances it was understood to be crucial. In Athens in the fifth century BC, a case brought to the law-courts alleged that a woman had poisoned her lover, Philoneus. In her defence she argued that she had intended to give him a drug to make him love her more, but had thought that increasing the dose would increase his love. Instead, Philoneus died instantly (ANTIPHON 1, *Prosecution of the Stepmother for Poisoning*, 19). It was widely recognised in classical Greece that certain drug substances could have beneficial effects – to relax the patient – or highly dangerous effects – even killing the patient – according to dosage, and it was acknowledged that the dividing line between low, moderate and high was very hard to determine.

Healing women

Drugs were particularly associated with women. Homer's epics feature Agamede, the daughter of King Augeas, who knew 'all the *pharmaka* of the earth' (HOMER, *Iliad* 11.739), and Helen of Troy who had a famous 'good drug' from Egypt, which made the drinker 'free from grief, free from anger, forgetting all sorrows' (HOMER, *Odyssey* 4.220–32). The effects of Homeric drugs are not always so good: the witch Circe also gave Odysseus' men a drug, but this made them forget their homes. Roman literature contains many examples of deliberate poisoning by women: it was claimed that the emperor Claudius had been poisoned by his wife Agrippina, aided by the famous female poisoner Locusta, and the doctor Xenophon (SUETONIUS, *Claudius* 44; TACITUS, Annals 12.66-7).

The Hippocratic texts in which most recipes for compound drugs appear are the three collections known as the *Gynaikeia*, or *Diseases of Women*. Only in these texts does the use of animal excrement as a drug feature, perhaps on the principle that applying something noxious would draw out the substance causing the symptoms, or perhaps because such excrement was regarded as a sort of 'fertiliser' for the womb, seen as a field in which the foetus would grow. The large number of recipes listed may mean that these gynaecological texts represent women's home remedies, traditionally handed down from mother to daughter, and here committed to writing for the first time. But we do not know whether this is the case and it is equally possible that the recipes were known to both sexes; perhaps the Hippocratic doctors also created some of their own, in keeping with their particular theories of causation and cure.

In later classical medicine many drug recipes are handed down to us with the names of their creator, in the format 'Recipe from Diocles, against toothache'. But by no means all are linked to famous doctors; others are attributed to boxing trainers, grooms, barbers and midwives.

In around 50-70 AD, Dioscorides, who came from what is now southern Turkey, produced the most famous materia medica of antiquity,

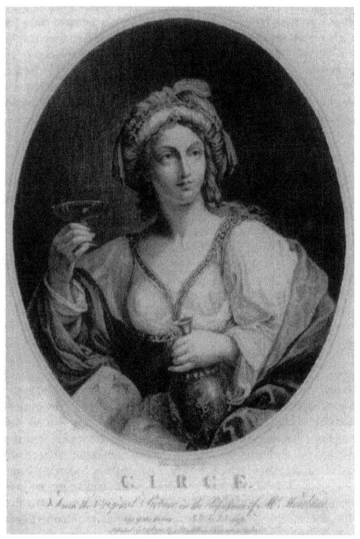

Fig 7 Circe with a goblet containing a drug. Engraving by W. Sharp, 1780.

based on many earlier books on the preparation of remedies which have now been lost. He classified over 1000 substances – mostly plants – according to the effects which individual drugs had on the body, but later editors rearranged the material into alphabetical order by substance name. Each plant is named, and its habitat and characteristics are described; he then gives the medical usages and side effects, and describes how to harvest, prepare and store the drug. He noted that plants have different effects depending on the soil in which they grow and the season at which they are harvested. He includes any uses of the plant in magic. Galen used Dioscorides, but reordered the classification into 'degrees' – a plant could be 'heating and drying in the fourth degree', for example, if it was in the most hot and dry category. The work of Dioscorides remained in use through the Middle Ages, when it was translated into Latin, Arabic and Armenian. After the invention of printing it was translated into many European languages, often with woodcut illustrations. These illustrations vary so widely that they do not necessarily help us to match the plants with those known today.

Efficacy

Western medicine had few effective drugs before the twentieth century. Pain-killers such as wine, opium and hemlock were known in the ancient world, but it was not until the sixteenth century that such drugs as the 'Jesuits' bark' (cinchona, used against fevers) and mercury (used to promote sweating in syphilis, but running the risk of gradually poisoning the patient) were used. The value of foxglove (digitalis) in heart failure was not known until the eighteenth century. But what counts as 'effective' is linked to the question of defining disease. In ancient humoral medicine illness could be a highly individual matter, relying on a particular combination of features unique to the patient. Although the phrasing 'a sickness takes hold of a patient' was also used, patients suffering from a condition with the same general name (such as gout, or dropsy) would usually not be treated in the same way as every other person with the same symptoms.

In some Hippocratic texts, such as *Diseases* 2, diseases are named, but in a very vague way, usually by the most prominent symptom: 'hiccupping disease', 'lethargy', 'withering disease' and 'belching disease'. Here the lists of remedies and dietary instructions are the same for everyone with that condition, although some conditions are stated as affecting particular groups; 'phlegmatic disease' affects more women than men (*Diseases* 2.70). In other texts, such as *Diseases of Women*, lists of remedies include many alternatives for one type of disturbance, given in the format 'If the womb causes pressure, a recipe...another one...or...' without any guidelines as to which should be selected. Individual factors could have been taken into account at this stage, especially since another section of *Diseases of Women* states that women should be given different treatment if they are old or young, and have a fair or a dark complexion.

More commonly, however, in classical humoral medicine a patient has an individual disturbance which needs to be treated by looking at his or her age, temperament, way of life and environment. In contrast, in modern medicine the same 'disease' is given the same treatment in all patients: the goal is 'a pill for every ill'.

The placebo effect?

What is known as 'the placebo effect', from the Latin for 'I will please', is accepted in modern medicine. Sometimes a substance which has no biochemical action will nevertheless make the patient feel better. The evidence suggests that simply taking a pill may have real, measurable effects on the body, even changing heart rate and blood pressure. Some studies have shown that capsules have a stronger placebo effect than tablets, and that coloured capsules are more effective than white ones. The author of the Hippocratic *Places in Man* 46 may be arguing against the placebo effect. He argues that medicine depends not on luck but on understanding. 'Real drugs' do not rely on luck to make the patient better, and substances which are 'not drugs', even if given with good luck, do not really cure the patient. For him, there is some power in the materials administered to the patient.

So, did ancient medicine 'work' by a placebo effect? Although some of the treatments used, such as rubbing fat or oil on to a sore area, would have eased suffering, many of the drugs given are more difficult to assess. There were certainly powerful herbs used, for example, in emetics and purges. Substances could rapidly produce a feeling of increased heat or coolness, and the patient would then wait for this effect to move through the body. But even substances which make no sense in modern terms would have had associations with myth and ritual. The explanations for symptoms given by the doctor would have reassured patients that there was some reason for why they felt so ill, and the careful attention to every aspect of their diet and way of life may have made them feel 'looked after'. Even the more unpleasant treatments may have helped, if the patient had faith in the doctor's methods.

Chapter 8
After ancient medicine

The ideas of Hippocrates and Galen formed the basis of medical education and treatment into the nineteenth century. The history of the transmission of the ancient medical texts is a complex one but even when few actual works of Hippocrates, the 'Father of medicine', and Galen, often known as the 'Prince of physicians', were available, they were still seen as the founders of medicine. However, their authority was gradually eroded from the sixteenth century onwards.

Translation and transmission

In the Greek-speaking East of the former Roman empire, Alexandria remained an important centre for medical education into the eighth century AD, and students there were expected to read Hippocratic and Galenic treatises. In the West there was less knowledge of these works, because few were translated into Latin before the eleventh century. In sixth-century Ravenna in Italy further new Latin translations of some Hippocratic texts were made, but the focus was on the more practical texts rather than on the theory behind the remedies.

Many theoretical Hippocratic treatises, and much of Galen's work, survived only in the Arab world, where ninth- and tenth-century rulers paid for translations to be made from Greek into Arabic. The Arab medical writers and translators included ar-Razi (Rhazes) in around 900 AD, and Ibn Sina (Avicenna) who was born in 980 AD. In the eleventh and twelfth centuries some of these works were then translated from Arabic into Latin, making them once more available to Western medicine. Meanwhile, during the twelfth and thirteenth centuries, new Latin translations were being made in Salerno in the south of Italy of some Greek medical texts, and a collection of Hippocratic, Galenic, Byzantine and Arabic medical writings was developed for teaching purposes. This collection, known as the *Articella*, went on to be used in many parts of Europe.

In the universities of medieval western Europe medicine was taught as part of 'natural philosophy', which held that God could best be known through his creation. From the second century AD onwards Christianity had included different approaches to medicine. Christ was seen as the

'Great Physician', who heals through prayer and faith and does not even charge a fee; some believed that really good Christians needed nothing more, particularly if much disease was the result of sin, making medical intervention less relevant than pilgrimage and repentance. Other Christian writers saw medicine as one of God's gifts to mortals, even if it was learned from pagan writers; Hippocrates could not be blamed for his paganism because he lived before Christ, while Galen was sometimes presented as a secret Christian.

The medieval Christian belief in God's revelation through creation was completely in keeping with the ideas not only of Galen but also of Aristotle, both of whom argued that anatomy could show the design in Nature. Pliny's claim that Nature has provided all the remedies we need could easily be merged with the idea that God has made provision for our health. Aristotle's methods of logical reasoning and rhetorical argument were also taught to university students. Galen's authority was unassailable in Western medicine from the twelfth century until the sixteenth century, when a range of challenges to his position emerged.

New texts and new diseases

One challenge came from the invention of the printing press: in the early sixteenth century a translation of the complete Hippocratic corpus from Greek into Latin was published. Although Galen had invariably referred to 'the divine Hippocrates', he himself was traditionally known, as already mentioned, as the 'Prince of Physicians'. But the preface to the Calvi translation of the Hippocratic corpus, published in 1525, described Hippocrates as 'without dispute, of all physicians, the Prince'. So, how was a doctor to react if the newly-available Hippocratic works contradicted the more familiar words of Galen: who was supreme? However, although it had now become possible for learned doctors, educated in universities, to read Hippocrates in Latin – the Greek language was still very little known in western Europe – they continued to see in the texts what Galen told them was there. They believed Galen's assessment of which Hippocratic texts were best and Galen's model of the body continued to guide their practice.

From the late fifteenth century, a number of diseases appeared which could not be found in the ancient medical writers; these included syphilis and the 'English sweat'. However, rather than thinking these new diseases made ancient medicine irrelevant, many scholars argued that the solution was to find better manuscripts of Hippocratic and Galenic treatises, or to discover previously unknown texts by these authors. New diseases stimulated the search for manuscripts all over Europe.

Travel outside Europe also challenged Galen. New plants were discovered which did not feature in Greek and Roman sources. Some scholars wanted to match them up with plants mentioned in Dioscorides but previously unidentified, while others tried to classify them as, for example, 'hot and dry in the second degree' so that they could be fitted into Galenic drug lore. People also began to wonder whether ancient medicine held all the answers when they were far away from their native land. In the seventeenth century English writers went even further, questioning whether classical remedies were appropriate outside the Mediterranean, or whether there should be 'English herbs for English people'. In art, new discoveries of classical sculpture made some people ask whether human bodies had changed so much since the heroic images of antiquity that ancient medicine no longer applied. For example, some writers believed that the amounts of blood taken in ancient bloodletting were more than a Renaissance body could bear.

Vesalius and human dissection

A further challenge came from the work of the great anatomist Andreas Vesalius (1514-64). He came from a medical family; his great-grandfather was city physician to Brussels, his grandfather wrote a commentary on the first four sections of *Aphorisms,* and his father was an apothecary to the Holy Roman Emperor Charles V. By the sixteenth century, human dissection – abandoned after Herophilus and Erasistratus – was again being practised. It was revived not to discover how the body worked but to give glory to God as the creator of human beings, seen as the peak of his creation.

In early fourteenth-century Italy, the medieval practice of performing autopsies on some saints' bodies, to reveal exceptional aspects of their anatomies – such as Christian symbols on their internal organs – was supplemented by human dissections, stimulated at first by lawyers needing to know the cause of death. Slowly, over the next 200 years, other parts of Europe took up the practice of dissection as an important part of a medical student's training, often using the bodies of criminals donated by the city in which the dissection took place. These performances were intended to prove that even the lowest criminal could demonstrate God's perfect design. A junior professor of medicine would read aloud from a book by an ancient authority – such as Galen – while a surgeon or butcher opened up the body, and a senior professor of medicine pointed out the relevant parts. Sixteenth-century drawings of anatomy theatres show packed audiences who could not possibly see the finer points of the demonstration, but whose presence was more like that of a congregation at a religious ceremony.

Vesalius graduated in medicine at Padua and rapidly established himself as an innovative anatomist. He claimed that the skills of the doctor, surgeon and apothecary, divided up in the Middle Ages, were once more united in one man: himself. Like Aristotle and Galen, he believed in comparative anatomy; like Galen, he performed frequent private dissections as well as public ones. In the illustrations of the human body in his *Six Anatomical Tables* (1538) Vesalius had mixed up human, ape and other animal features, still representing the arteries and the veins as separate systems, as Galen had done. In Table 3 he showed the *rete mirabile*, a network of veins at the base of the brain in some ruminant animals, which Galen had wrongly supposed existed in humans. In 1543, at the age of 28, he published *The Fabric of the Human Body*. He still made what we now recognise as errors. For example, he agreed with Galen that blood moved from the right side of the heart to the left through 'invisible pores' in the thick dividing wall of the heart; however, no such pores exist. But Vesalius himself identified over 200 errors he had found in Galen, many of them due to Galen having failed to understand the differences between human and animal anatomy; he said that Galen was 'deceived by his apes'.

However, beneath this attack, Vesalius still worked in the Galenic tradition, despite his emphasis on 'autopsy', or seeing for oneself. He followed the order of argument of Galen's great anatomy text *On Anatomical Procedures*, the seven Books of *The Fabric of the Human Body* covering the bones, muscles, veins, arteries, abdomen, thorax and head. Lost to the Middle Ages, this treatise had been rediscovered a few years before Vesalius published his work. When he was invited to dissect in Bologna in 1540 he had also started with the bones, bringing with him a skeleton, so that he could keep referring to the structure of the body as his dissection progressed. This was exactly what Galen had recommended. By carrying out human dissection, in addition to animal dissection and vivisection, he saw himself as continuing Galen's work.

Chemical medicine

Further attacks on Galen came from the work of Paracelsus (c.1493-1541) and his followers. There is no evidence that Paracelsus took a medical degree, and he claimed that the best way to learn was not from a university but through travel. He believed in speaking to all types of people to see what they could teach him: these included barbers, bathkeepers, learned physicians, women, magicians and alchemists. He was briefly city physician in Basle, where he lectured on medicine in German rather than the usual Latin, attacked the classical authorities and argued that experience was better than books: he is famous for burning one of the classics of Arabic medicine, Avicenna's *Canon*, in 1527.

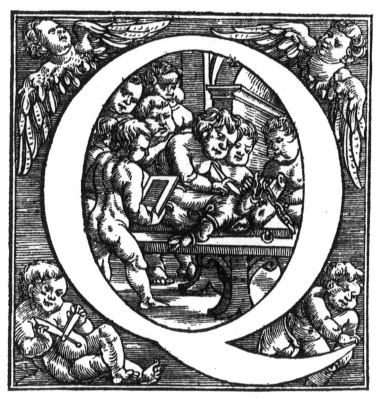

Fig 8 Cherubs vivisect a pig; initial 'Q' from Vesalius' *Fabrica*. It was assumed that knowledge gained from animals could be applied to humans.

He abandoned the theory of the four humours and argued that the basis of the body was the chemical process of distillation, in which burning and mixing separated out the pure essence. He proposed that there were three principles in the body: sulphur, mercury and salt. A disease is an 'entity' coming into the body and invading man's 'castle of health', and moving to a location in the body where it lodges. Treatment should be aimed at the 'entity', rather than treating the whole body. He thought that the natural world contained clues on which plant is best for which disease; for example, thistle pricks so it is good for internal prickling feelings. But he also used minerals and metals to cure disease and believed that even poisons, if properly prepared, could cure.

Another sixteenth-century writer who thought that disease came from outside the body was Fracastoro, who described 'the seeds of disease'. However, he worked within the framework of humoral medicine and miasma theory, so his ideas did not appear as threatening to traditional medicine as those of Paracelsus.

The Scientific Revolution

The seventeenth century experienced what has been called a 'Scientific Revolution'. Debates took place all over Europe between learned individuals from different subject areas: in England the Royal Society received its charter in 1662. They agreed that the world could be understood by careful observation, trusting the senses but also developing new instruments to enhance them, such as the telescope and microscope. The new science was experimental science: it was believed that you could repeat an experiment and get the same result every time, because the world is predictable and the mathematical laws by which it works can be discovered by human knowledge, divided into separate sciences. Many writers thought that the world – and the human body – functions in a predictable and rational way, like a machine. By the nineteenth century, after the introduction of anaesthesia in the 1840s, surgery was seen as the best way to mend the machine, simply opening up the body and repairing the defective parts.

In the seventeenth century van Helmont (1579-1644), who saw chemical changes in the body as responsible for processes such as digestion, argued that new diseases are created by God, while old ones change to become more serious, so that new ways of healing must continue to be discovered, 'For the Art grows every day'. New diseases meant a challenge to the Galenic model of disease. Experiments on air by, among others, Robert Boyle (1627-91), showed its role in sustaining life and led to a rethinking of Galen's idea that the lungs worked simply to 'cool down' the heart. Galen's view of the body was further undermined by William Harvey's discovery of the circulation of the blood – published in 1628 – which showed that the veins and arteries did not form separate systems, but were part of one network through which the blood moved from the heart and back to it again.

A greater focus on drugs, rather than diet, as the basis of medicine was found in the work of van Helmont. He agreed with Paracelsus that a disease was a 'thing', and his interest in finding the right drug for each condition was reinforced by what has been called the 'medical market-place' of this period. Drugs were literally sold in the markets, by quacks who lacked any university training. These quacks mixed up traditional and new ideas, but had in common a claim that the same drug will cure everyone with the same condition. This sort of medicine was much cheaper than hiring a traditional Galenic healer who would need to know all about the patient's constitution and life, and would then give instructions on how to modify every aspect; for Galen, every drug needed to be considered in relation to the individual nature of the patient being treated.

However, the new science did not always question Galen. From the seventeenth century onwards microscopes were used, and researchers found they could see 'little worms' in the blood. Their use actually encouraged the idea of 'invisible structures' at an even smaller size, which only a better microscope would make visible. It was thought that the senses were not enough; that there is 'a world beneath our senses'. Galen's 'invisible pores' in the heart were at least theoretically possible, and Harvey's discovery of the circulation of the blood depended on a belief in 'capillaries' linking the arteries to the veins; these capillaries could not actually be seen by Harvey but, with better microscopy, they would later become visible.

Other changes in the eighteenth century meant that Galen's view, that the best doctor is also a philosopher, was disputed. In 1701 the great medical teacher Herman Boerhaave (1668-1738), who taught the theory of medicine, botany, clinical medicine and chemistry at Leiden, believed that the best medicine was that which followed Hippocrates in every particular. By 1703, however, he recommended instead reading the works of writers on mechanics and physics, such as Isaac Newton. Boerhaave used a hydraulic model of the body in which anatomical structures acted like pulleys, levers and bellows. He argued that doctors should not discuss the soul, or the nature of life; medicine should not concern itself with the secondary, underlying causes. Many writers of this period believed that anatomy was not the key to medicine, as Galen had suggested; they argued that increasingly detailed knowledge of anatomy did not improve the treatment of patients.

Modern medicine

The death of Galenism was also caused by technology. In the eighteenth century it became possible to quantify the pulse, giving a number rather than talking about strong, erratic, or crawling pulses. By the nineteenth century, a range of instruments shifted the focus further from the doctor's use of the five senses to the neutrality of numbers. These included the stethoscope (1816), the thermometer (1860s) and various methods of blood testing – for example, Gowers' haemocytometer (1877) made it easier to count the number of red blood cells in a sample. As medicine relied on the laboratory, the role of the doctor shifted. The home visit was replaced not just with the trip to the doctor's surgery, but also by reliance on the hospital to give the results of tests for the doctor to interpret.

Germ theory meant that many diseases could be seen – literally, with increasingly sophisticated microscopes – as caused by invading organisms rather than as internal disturbances. In the seventeenth century Antoni van Leeuwenhoek (1632-1723) had observed 'little animals' in water. In the nineteenth century the connection between specific bacteria and specific diseases was finally proved. Even newer ways of seeing the body, from X-rays (1895) – which show bone – to the CAT scanner and MRI scanner which show soft tissues, meant that the presence of a tumour or other lesion could be recognised objectively, rather than assumed from external signs or from touching the body.

Improved public health and treatment by antibiotics mean that the 'fevers' – acute infections – which were the major diseases of the past have been replaced by chronic degenerative diseases such as heart disease and arthritis. Knowledge of diet, and of the roles of vitamins and minerals, has virtually eliminated the 'deficiency diseases' in the developed world. The part played in various bodily processes by hormones (from the Greek verb to excite or arouse) has been clarified. The Human Genome Project has succeeded in mapping the genes.

Plato and Galen would approve: modern medicine is centred on drugs, even if they are now made from synthetic compounds rather than from the plants provided by nature. Willow bark was used in the eighteenth century to reduce fever and pain; in the second half of the nineteenth century it was synthesised in the laboratory, and tested on animals and people. At the turn of the century the synthetic compound was named 'Aspirin'. Many drugs from this period were discovered by testing the by-products of chemical manufacture. New 'designer drugs' are now created in order to target particular conditions. For many centuries mental illness was treated by the same methods of blood-letting and purging used for bodily disorders. From the late eighteenth century onwards treatment of the mad ranged from 'restraint', where a person was put in manacles or in a strait-jacket to control them, to 'moral therapy' where the insane were treated gently, like children, and the doctor waited for them to improve. In the twentieth century electricity and surgery were used on the mentally ill but, after 1950, the ascendancy of drug treatment also affected this area, with new drugs being used to stabilise patients.

As medicine has advanced, so our expectations of medicine have also risen; we consult our doctors more and more, and we expect to feel better quickly. At the same time, our faith in 'a pill for every ill' is being challenged by drug-resistant microbes, drug side-effects (such as the tragedy of thalidomide) and increased pressure on medical spending by governments. We expect to have the latest tests performed and we expect medicine to continue to conquer disease. But we also expect doctors to offer us the personal care, and the understanding of us as individuals, which were appropriate to an earlier era of medicine.

Conclusion

This introduction to Greek and Roman medicine has suggested many areas in which similarities exist between classical views of disease and healing, and ideas still found today. This may not be surprising, since we share not only a common experience of the human body – its growth, its failings and its eventual death – but also a cultural and artistic heritage. Like the Greeks and Romans, we think that some diseases come from 'outside' even if germs have, to a large extent, replaced gods. Like them, we see other diseases as arising inside our bodies, making it our own responsibility to balance our humours, or to ensure the correct intake of protein or fibre. We share a belief that the environment in which we live and work can affect our health, and that climate can influence our well-being. We also share a belief in doctors: experts to help us make sense of some of the things our bodies do, and to reassure us that our individual symptoms can be reinterpreted as part of a pattern which other people, too, have experienced. Modern anatomical knowledge and medical terminology can be traced back directly to the Greeks, although developments in medical technology, pathology, microbiology and genetics have made methods of diagnosis and treatment very different. In addition, we share anxieties about the risks of entrusting our bodies to a doctor's care.

Neither we nor the ancients can explain everything. For the ancient Greeks diseases could be sent and cured by the gods, but Hesiod's myth of Pandora's jar also suggests that some diseases are free agents, wandering the world outside the control of Zeus. Disease was unpredictable, and to be feared. Ancient medical writers tried to find ways to forecast the course of disease – using prognostic signs and critical days – to restore the balance of humours and to remove obstacles to their proper flow.

Today, when the origins of disease are often better understood, the old questions still need to be answered. If many diseases come from germs, why do some people catch them while others remain healthy? Why does the same disease kill one person but only affect another in a mild form? In the eighteenth century there was a renewed emphasis on lifestyle and personal morality as responsible for such variation; by the beginning of the twentieth century the concept of immunity was being explored, and ways of giving people immunity were developed for some diseases using vaccines and 'anti-toxins'. But at the same time a culture of 'healthy living' has developed, in which we are bombarded through the media with information about how much fruit we should eat, water we should drink and exercise we should take. Alongside scientific medicine, older ideas about personal responsibility for health continue to exist.

Because we still need to feel that we are in control of our world, new diseases present a huge threat to our collective sense of confidence. Where medicine appears to have failed, other types of explanation can be tried. Early attempts to see AIDS as God's punishment for sexual licence recall many other occasions in history when a new and apparently inexplicable disease has been attributed by some contemporaries to divine agency: most notably, the arrival of syphilis in Europe at the end of the fifteenth century, but also the plague which hit Athens from 430 BC onwards. Both the medicine of the ancient Mediterranean and modern medicine come up against similar problems of meaning and explanation.

Those who perform medicine – mostly, doctors – are very different in some ways, as their role is now that of state-funded, trained and licensed practitioners. For the classical world our evidence is skewed by accidents of survival of the sources, giving us very detailed knowledge of one exceptional doctor – Galen – with a shortage of information on what else was on offer. While we can glimpse the root-cutters and diviners, they have not left us the mass of written information we have on Hippocratic and Galenic medicine. Greek rural medicine may have been much like the medicine of rural Italy; most evidence survives for urban medicine, but we can still glimpse family-based healing and nursing care in both the Greek and Roman worlds. Today, too, the doctor is neither the first line of assistance nor the only option available to us.

In much of this book, I have emphasised the individual: the lone doctor, trying to prove his skills by his persuasive rhetoric, modest clothing, clever theories and impressive treatment. However, not only were such doctors organised into family groups and guilds: the state also played a role in ancient medicine. State support may have been behind the work of the Alexandrian anatomists, who performed human dissection with the agreement of the ruling Ptolemies. Although the Greek doctor Archagathus may have been welcomed by the Roman state at a time of war, his transformation from being a valued 'wound-doctor' to becoming a feared 'butcher' may suggest something else: deeply ingrained misunderstandings between Greeks and Romans as to what medicine was about.

Both of these examples – Greek medicine in Egypt and Greek medicine at Rome – can suggest the importance of the social context within which ideas exist. If the (Roman) patient has different ideas about how the body works and what 'healing' is supposed to consist of, then what the (Greek) doctor says may not make sense; not believing the explanation for the symptoms, the patient is less likely to follow the treatment. Medical anthropology in modern western society has shown that doctors today play along with patients' beliefs, phrasing their explanations for illness in terms of unscientific popular ideas such as 'feed a cold, starve a fever', which implies that 'colds' are due to a failure to look after oneself properly, while 'fevers' are the result of invading organisms which need to be deprived of food so that they will die. Doctors need to express themselves in a way that patients will understand. The gap between 'medical' knowledge and 'lay' knowledge in the ancient world was, however, far smaller than today; the works of Pliny and Celsus show how much an elite male Roman was supposed to know about medicine.

Medicine has moved away from everyday knowledge as part of the process of becoming a science; where ancient medicine was very closely based on the senses, modern medicine looks to the laboratory for truth. Yet medicine also remains an art, in which the doctor needs to persuade the patient of his or her skills. It is possible that the personality of the healer is the strongest placebo of all. In the Hippocratic texts on self-presentation, what matters is to act like a 'gentleman': although the modern hospital uniform of the white coat and stethoscope is more concerned with impressing upon the patient the scientific nature of modern medicine, specialists and general practitioners alike need to persuade the patient of their trustworthiness and sympathy as well as their knowledge.

An emphasis on the importance of the healer may, however, be more about rejecting patients' attempts to heal themselves. As we saw in Chapter 5, Cato – who believed in self-help within the family – claimed that the efficacy of cabbage lay in the plant itself, perhaps contrasting its use to remedies where a chant accompanied a drug. This would suggest that you do not need a doctor to use cabbage successfully. In contrast, according to Galen, Herophilus had earlier claimed that a drug substance was nothing without the person who knew how to use it (*On the Composition of Drugs according to Place* 6.8).

That person is clearly the product of society and culture. The surviving texts of Hippocratic medicine include some from a very early stage of Greek literacy, where lists were made, connections noticed and theories developed to account for observed patterns. The patterns which were observed were 'seen' because they made sense in terms of pre-existing ideas: about the nature of the universe, the differences between women and men, and the ritual significance of certain numbers. They drew heavily on analogies with the natural world of agriculture and cookery, whereas eighteenth-century medicine looked to the world of machines.

The task of medicine remains constant: to explain why people feel ill and to make them feel better. Its methods may change, but practitioners still need to establish their authority, gain the trust of the patient, and tell a story which accounts for the symptoms and promises hope.

Suggestions for Further Study

1. Can we distinguish between 'medicine' and 'magic'? What would be our criteria? Do they use words and objects in different ways? Is it more a question of the person doing the action, the reasons they give, the methods they use, or the results they achieve?

2. How did Greeks and Romans explain disease? Whose fault is it? How would a patient and his/her family react to doctors' explanations? What treatments would follow from different explanations and would some be less painful or difficult than others?

3. Hippocratic authors often use an emphatic first person – 'But *I* tell patients to do this....' – in a way that hints at a lost body of medical and other texts giving different views. How far can we reconstruct the ideas of those against whom the Hippocratics were arguing? What ideas do the Hippocratics most strongly reject? What sort of healers would have held these ideas?

4. What skills did a Greek or Roman doctor need? How far do these differ from the skills of modern doctors? To what extent did they rely on the evidence of their senses?

5. In what ways have later developments in medicine influenced the way we understand ancient medical texts? How can we avoid seeing ancient medicine through modern eyes? What are the dangers of applying modern diagnoses to ancient disease descriptions? Modern medical journals still feature articles on the correct 'diagnosis' of the Athenian plague. Does this really matter?

6. Why has Hippocrates been seen as the 'father of alternative medicine'?

7. Is medicine only something which doctors do? How separate were the doctor's and the patient's knowledge of the body in the ancient world? What are the effects of modern scientific medicine moving away from everyday language and knowledge?

8. What is the best way of understanding how the body works? Is the western focus on anatomy really justified, or did ancient writers who complained that it did not help in understanding disease have a point?

9. How has the relationship between religion and medicine changed over time? Why have these changes occurred? Does medicine always need religion to explain why particular individuals are struck by disease?

10. How do we control the behaviour of doctors today? How does this differ from the situation in the ancient world?

11. Was medicine before the twentieth century 'generally some pretty ineffectual drugs washed down with a hefty gulp of the placebo effect' (R. Porter)?

Suggestions for Further Reading

Original sources in translation

The Loeb Classical Library currently includes 8 volumes of the Hippocratic corpus, giving the Greek text with English translation.

Lloyd, G.E.R., *Hippocratic Writings* (Penguin, 1978) is indispensable; it includes a good selection of texts.

Longrigg, J., *Greek Medicine from the Heroic to the Hellenistic Age* (Duckworth, 1998): a very wide range of sources are translated, including sources from ancient Egypt and the Near East, and are also discussed at length; however, they are used to illustrate a very personal argument about how the Greeks developed 'rational' medicine.

Brock A.J. (tr.), *Greek Medicine, being Extracts Illustrative of Medical Writers from Hippocrates to Galen* (J.M. Dent and Sons, 1929; reprinted AMS Press, 1977). Still a useful collection of sources, covering much of ancient medicine; selections from the Alexandrians are included.

Von Staden, H., *Herophilus: the Art of Medicine in Early Alexandria* (Cambridge, 1989). The complete edition of those fragments of Herophilus' work so far identified; this magisterial work contains excellent discussions of the context and content of the Alexandrian anatomists.

Nutton, V. (ed and tr. with commentary), *Galen, On Prognosis* (Berlin, 1979): Galen's account of how he made his mark on Roman medicine reads almost like a novel.

Singer, P.N., *Selected Works: Galen* (Oxford University Press, 1997).

Grant, M., *Galen on Diet* (Routledge, 2000): these two collections make a range of Galen's works easily available. Singer's book has a particularly good introductory section.

Modern historical works

Conrad, L.I. et al., *The Western Medical Tradition 800 BC - AD 1800* (Cambridge University Press, 1995): a very good general survey of the period, including three chapters on the Greek and Roman worlds, with a full bibliography.

Porter, R. (ed.), *Cambridge Illustrated History of Medicine* (Cambridge University Press, 1996): goes from antiquity up to the present day; thoughtful essays broken up by short sections summarising key events, theories and individuals.

Rihll, T., *Greek Science* (Oxford University Press, 1999): concise and enjoyable survey with a chapter on 'Biology and Medicine'.

Jouanna, J., *Hippocrates* (Johns Hopkins University Press, 1999): full discussion of the Hippocratic texts, the role of ancient physicians and the place of Hippocratic medicine in Greek culture; includes a summary of the later fortunes of Hippocratic ideas.

Grmek, M.D., *Diseases in the Ancient Greek World* (Baltimore, 1989): a detailed account from the perspective of a wide-ranging medical historian.

Majno, G., *The Healing Hand: Man and Wound in the Ancient World* (Cambridge, MA, 1981). This work compares the classical Mediterranean with early Indian and Chinese medicine; it also reconstructs ancient experiments and analyses ancient remedies.

Jackson, R., *Doctors and Diseases in the Roman Empire* (British Museum Press, 1988): covering more geographically and chronologically than the title suggests, this is a thorough, well-illustrated account with plenty of information on the archaeological evidence.

Swain, S., *Hellenism and Empire: Language, Classicism, and Power in the Greek World AD 50-250* (Clarendon Press, 1996): chapter 11 provides a very useful summary of Galen's life and work within its social context.

Lloyd, G.E.R., *Magic, Reason and Experience* (BCP, 1999) and *Science, Folklore and Ideology* (BCP, 1999): these highly influential works examine the social and cultural background to early Greek science and medicine.

Dean-Jones, L., *Women's Bodies in Classical Greek Science* (Clarendon Press, 1994) focuses in particular on comparing views on women and their treatment found in Hippocrates and Aristotle, while King, H., *Hippocrates' Woman: Reading the Female Body in Ancient Greece* (Routledge, 1998) concentrates on how ancient Greek ideas about women were used and re-used in the history of medicine.

The following works are recommended for those who would like to think about the later uses of ancient medicine:

Rothman, D.J., Marcus, S. and Kiceluk, S.A. (eds), *Medicine and Western civilization* (New Brunswick, NJ, 1995): a sourcebook which covers a wide period and includes a very good selection of passages with some commentary.

Siraisi, N., *Medieval and Early Renaissance Medicine* (Chicago University Press, 1990).

Lindemann, M., *Medicine and Society in Early Modern Europe* (Cambridge University Press, 1999).

Porter, R., *The Greatest Benefit to Mankind* (HarperCollins, 1999).

Index